Essential MCQs

Surgical Finals

D0314340

Essential MCQs

for Surgical Finals

Delilah Hassanally MSc FRCS (Eng)

Specialist Registrar in General Surgery
North East Thames

Rema Kaur Wasan BA MBBS MA MRCP FRCR

Consultant Radiologist
King's College Hospital
London

© 2003 PASTEST LTD
Egerton Court
Parkgate Estate
Knutsford
Cheshire WA16 8DX

Telephone: 01565 752000

First published 1997
Reprinted 1999, 2001, 2003
Second edition 2003

ISBN 1 901198 15 4

A catalogue record for this book is available from the British Library.

The information contained within this book was obtained by the authors from reliable sources. However, while every effort has been made to ensure its accuracy, no responsibility for loss, damage or injury occasioned to any person acting or refraining from action as a result of information contained herein can be accepted by the publisher or authors.

PasTest Revision Books and Intensive Courses
PasTest has been established in the field of postgraduate medical education since 1972, providing revision books and intensive study courses for doctors preparing for their professional examinations.
Books and courses are available for the following specialties:
MRCP Part 1 and Part 2, MRCPCH Part 1 and Part 2, MRCS, MRCOG, MRCGP, DRCOG, MRCPsych, DCH, FRCA and PLAB.
For further details contact:
PasTest, Freepost, Knutsford, Cheshire WA16 7BR
Tel: 01565 752000   Fax: 01565 650264
E-mail: enquiries@pastest.co.uk
Web site: www.pastest.co.uk

Typeset by Breeze Limited, Manchester.
Printed by MPG Books Limited, Bodmin, Cornwall.

CONTENTS

INTRODUCTION

There are many multiple choice question books for postgraduate medical examinations, and for years undergraduates preparing for finals have been forced to struggle with these as there is very little revision material specific to their needs.

The aim of this book is to provide 'real' MCQ practice examinations at the appropriate level for undergraduates sitting their final surgical examinations. These questions will also benefit those sitting the PLAB examination.

This book contains three test papers designed to be similar in format, content and balance of subjects to surgical finals MCQ examinations. Answers and detailed teaching notes are given for each question. The questions are as 'real' as possible; they include material that has been remembered by medical students after their surgical finals examinations.

There is a natural tendency to recall the harder and more confusing topics, but rather than avoiding these, we have deliberately included them and so the pass mark for each paper is probably a little less than 50%. We hope medical students will use this to their advantage; everyone will get the easy questions right, but the medical student who enters the examination having done the more difficult questions should not just pass, but pass well.

The second edition contains extra questions to cover recent developments. In addition, we have revised questions according to changes in current medical opinion and to reflect changes in examination emphasis.

Delilah Hassanally
Rema Wasan

MCQ EXAMINATION TECHNIQUE

Before sitting an MCQ examination, you will need to know how many questions are likely to be on the paper and how long you will be given to complete it. Thus you will be able to assess the approximate amount of time that can be spent on each question. Pacing yourself accurately during the examination to finish on time, or with time to spare, is essential.

In MCQ examinations you must read the question (both stem and items A–E) carefully. Take care not to mark the wrong boxes and think very carefully before making a mark on the answer sheet. Regard each option as being independent of every other item – each refers to a specific quantum of knowledge. The item (or the stem and the item taken together) make up a statement. You are required to indicate whether you regard this statement as 'True' or 'False'. Look only at a single statement when answering – disregard all the other statements presented in the question. They have nothing to do with the item you are concentrating on. Any of the statements may be true or false; sometimes none of the stem answers are true.

As you go through the questions, you can either mark your answers immediately on the answer sheet, or you can mark them on the question paper and then transfer them to the answer sheet. If you adopt the second approach, you must take great care not to make any errors and not to run out of time, since you will not be allowed extra time to transfer marks to the answer sheet. The answer sheet must always be marked neatly and carefully according to the instructions given. Careless marking is probably one of the commonest causes of rejection of answer sheets by the document reader.

- Do as many good quality practice papers as possible. This will help you to identify your strengths and weaknesses in time for further study. You can also use the Revision Index at the back of this book to find questions on specific topics, so that after you have done some reading you can test your knowledge.

- With the three exams provided in this book be strict with yourself and work under realistic exam conditions. You should develop an understanding of your own work rate so that you know how much time you can spend on each question.

- Read each question several times. Nobody at this vital stage in their career should be wasting marks because they misread or misunderstood the question.

- Each exam in this book contains 60 questions.

- If you have to guess the answer to a question, put a special mark next to it. You will then be able to find out if you are a good guesser. This is especially important if your examination is negatively marked, ie marks will be deducted for incorrect answers. It is important to know what you know as well as what you don't know.

- Use the Revision Checklist on the following pages to keep a record of the subjects you have covered and feel confident about. This will ensure that you do not miss out any key topics.

SAMPLE ANSWER SHEET

UNIVERSITY OF LONDON Management Systems Division

MULTIPLE-CHOICE EXAMINATION ANSWER SHEET

DATE..................

SURNAME...............

FIRST NAME(S)..............

Instructions: Use the HB pencil provided. To make an answer draw a single horizontal line along the dotted line above the appropriate letter or number. To answer 'TRUE' draw your line above the capital letter in the upper row. To answer 'FALSE' draw your line above the lower case letter in the lower row. For example:

[A] for 'TRUE'   [A] for 'FALSE'
[a]   [a]

If you change your mind and wish to cancel a completed answer, draw another line below the letter or number, along the dotted line. Do not rub out.

Candidate No.	Test No.	College No.
|0| |0| |0| |0|	|0| |0| |0| |0|	|0| |0|
|1| |1| |1| |1|	|1| |1| |1| |1|	|1| |1|
|2| |2| |2| |2|	|P| |2| |2| |2|	|2| |2|
|3| |3| |3| |3|	|3| |3| |3|	|3| |3|
|4| |4| |4| |4|	|4| |4| |4|	|4| |4|
|5| |5| |5| |5|	|5| |5| |5|	|5| |5|
|6| |6| |6| |6|	|6| |6| |6|	|6| |6|
|7| |7| |7| |7|	|7| |7| |7|	|7| |7|
|8| |8| |8| |8|	|8| |8| |8|	|8| |8|
|9| |9| |9| |9|	|9| |9| |9|	|9| |9|

Shown below is the correct method of completion, the correct method of cancellation/alteration and examples of various incorrect methods of completion.

CORRECT METHOD OF COMPLETION

True = [A]   False = [A]
       [a]   [a]

CORRECT METHOD OF CANCELLATION/ ALTERATION

To cancel a response, draw a line below the letter. Do not rub out. Thus:

[A] or [A] = Cancelled
[a]   [B]

To alter a response, first cancel. Then draw a line above the other letter. Thus:

False = [A]   True = [A]
        [a]   [a]

INCORRECT METHODS OF COMPLETION

Too faint [A]

Slanted [A]

Too low [A]

Too high [A]

Into box [A] [B]

Too short [A] [A] [A]

Isolated cancellation [A]

DETERMINATE TYPE T

1	[A] [B] [C] [D] [E] / [a] [b] [c] [d] [e]	13 [A] [B] [C] [D] [E] / [a] [b] [c] [d] [e]	25 [A] [B] [C] [D] [E] / [a] [b] [c] [d] [e]	37 [A] [B] [C] [D] [E] / [a] [b] [c] [d] [e]	49 [A] [B] [C] [D] [E] / [a] [b] [c] [d] [e]
2	[A] [B] [C] [D] [E] / [a] [b] [c] [d] [e]	14 [A] [B] [C] [D] [E] / [a] [b] [c] [d] [e]	26 [A] [B] [C] [D] [E] / [a] [b] [c] [d] [e]	38 [A] [B] [C] [D] [E] / [a] [b] [c] [d] [e]	50 [A] [B] [C] [D] [E] / [a] [b] [c] [d] [e]
3	[A] [B] [C] [D] [E] / [a] [b] [c] [d] [e]	15 [A] [B] [C] [D] [E] / [a] [b] [c] [d] [e]	27 [A] [B] [C] [D] [E] / [a] [b] [c] [d] [e]	39 [A] [B] [C] [D] [E] / [a] [b] [c] [d] [e]	51 [A] [B] [C] [D] [E] / [a] [b] [c] [d] [e]
4	[A] [B] [C] [D] [E] / [a] [b] [c] [d] [e]	16 [A] [B] [C] [D] [E] / [a] [b] [c] [d] [e]	28 [A] [B] [C] [D] [E] / [a] [b] [c] [d] [e]	40 [A] [B] [C] [D] [E] / [a] [b] [c] [d] [e]	52 [A] [B] [C] [D] [E] / [a] [b] [c] [d] [e]
5	[A] [B] [C] [D] [E] / [a] [b] [c] [d] [e]	17 [A] [B] [C] [D] [E] / [a] [b] [c] [d] [e]	29 [A] [B] [C] [D] [E] / [a] [b] [c] [d] [e]	41 [A] [B] [C] [D] [E] / [a] [b] [c] [d] [e]	53 [A] [B] [C] [D] [E] / [a] [b] [c] [d] [e]
6	[A] [B] [C] [D] [E] / [a] [b] [c] [d] [e]	18 [A] [B] [C] [D] [E] / [a] [b] [c] [d] [e]	30 [A] [B] [C] [D] [E] / [a] [b] [c] [d] [e]	42 [A] [B] [C] [D] [E] / [a] [b] [c] [d] [e]	54 [A] [B] [C] [D] [E] / [a] [b] [c] [d] [e]
7	[A] [B] [C] [D] [E] / [a] [b] [c] [d] [e]	19 [A] [B] [C] [D] [E] / [a] [b] [c] [d] [e]	31 [A] [B] [C] [D] [E] / [a] [b] [c] [d] [e]	43 [A] [B] [C] [D] [E] / [a] [b] [c] [d] [e]	55 [A] [B] [C] [D] [E] / [a] [b] [c] [d] [e]
8	[A] [B] [C] [D] [E] / [a] [b] [c] [d] [e]	20 [A] [B] [C] [D] [E] / [a] [b] [c] [d] [e]	32 [A] [B] [C] [D] [E] / [a] [b] [c] [d] [e]	44 [A] [B] [C] [D] [E] / [a] [b] [c] [d] [e]	56 [A] [B] [C] [D] [E] / [a] [b] [c] [d] [e]
9	[A] [B] [C] [D] [E] / [a] [b] [c] [d] [e]	21 [A] [B] [C] [D] [E] / [a] [b] [c] [d] [e]	33 [A] [B] [C] [D] [E] / [a] [b] [c] [d] [e]	45 [A] [B] [C] [D] [E] / [a] [b] [c] [d] [e]	57 [A] [B] [C] [D] [E] / [a] [b] [c] [d] [e]
10	[A] [B] [C] [D] [E] / [a] [b] [c] [d] [e]	22 [A] [B] [C] [D] [E] / [a] [b] [c] [d] [e]	34 [A] [B] [C] [D] [E] / [a] [b] [c] [d] [e]	46 [A] [B] [C] [D] [E] / [a] [b] [c] [d] [e]	58 [A] [B] [C] [D] [E] / [a] [b] [c] [d] [e]
11	[A] [B] [C] [D] [E] / [a] [b] [c] [d] [e]	23 [A] [B] [C] [D] [E] / [a] [b] [c] [d] [e]	35 [A] [B] [C] [D] [E] / [a] [b] [c] [d] [e]	47 [A] [B] [C] [D] [E] / [a] [b] [c] [d] [e]	59 [A] [B] [C] [D] [E] / [a] [b] [c] [d] [e]
12	[A] [B] [C] [D] [E] / [a] [b] [c] [d] [e]	24 [A] [B] [C] [D] [E] / [a] [b] [c] [d] [e]	36 [A] [B] [C] [D] [E] / [a] [b] [c] [d] [e]	48 [A] [B] [C] [D] [E] / [a] [b] [c] [d] [e]	60 [A] [B] [C] [D] [E] / [a] [b] [c] [d] [e]

Reproduced by kind permission of the University of London.

REVISION CHECKLIST

Use this checklist to record your revision progress. Tick the subjects when you feel confident that you have covered them adequately. This will ensure that you do not forget to revise any key topics. This list is arranged in approximate order of importance. Items closest to the top of each list are most likely to come up in examinations.

GASTROINTESTINAL SYSTEM – UPPER
- ❏ Acid reflux
- ❏ Peptic ulcer
- ❏ Achalasia
- ❏ Upper gastrointestinal bleed
- ❏ Small bowel obstruction
- ❏ Mesenteric embolus
- ❏ Crohn's disease
- ❏ Post-gastrectomy symptoms
- ❏ Oesophageal malignancy
- ❏ Paralytic ileus
- ❏ Pancreatitis; pancreatic tumours
- ❏ Acute appendicitis
- ❏ Hernias – femoral and inguinal
- ❏ Parotid tumours
- ❏ Carcinoma of the tongue
- ❏ Barium studies; endoscopy

GASTROINTESTINAL SYSTEM – LOWER
- ❏ Inflammatory bowel disease
- ❏ Diverticular disease
- ❏ Malignancy
- ❏ Fistulae
- ❏ Haemorrhoids
- ❏ Anal fissure
- ❏ Pilonidal abscess

HEPATOBILIARY SYSTEM
- ❏ Gallstones
- ❏ Cholecystitis
- ❏ Ascending cholangitis
- ❏ Jaundice
- ❏ Radiological procedures, eg, ERCP, PTC
- ❏ Hepatitis B
- ❏ Hydatid cyst of the liver

VASCULAR
Venous
- ❏ varicose veins
- ❏ deep vein thrombosis

Arterial
- ❏ ischaemia
- ❏ carotid stenosis
- ❏ peripheral vascular disease

RENAL SYSTEM
- ❏ Neoplasia
- ❏ Calculi
- ❏ Acute renal failure
- ❏ Investigations, eg, intravenous urography

UROGENITAL TRACT
- ❏ Testicular tumours
- ❏ Scrotal swellings
- ❏ Varicocele
- ❏ Hydrocele
- ❏ Undescended testes

TRAUMA
- ❏ Chest
- ❏ Spleen
- ❏ Kidney
- ❏ Head

SKIN
- ❏ Malignant melanoma
- ❏ Carbuncle
- ❏ Basal cell carcinoma

NERVOUS SYSTEM
- ❑ Horner's syndrome
- ❑ Bell's palsy

MISCELLANEOUS
- ❑ Breast – benign and malignant lesions
- ❑ Thyroid – cystic and solid swellings
- ❑ Post-operative complications
- ❑ Wound healing
- ❑ Fluid replacement
- ❑ Shock/hypovolaemia

OPERATIONS CHECKLIST

Medical students need to be aware of certain operations which are performed routinely. This short list is by no means comprehensive, but can be used as a guideline. You need to know the indication for the operation and basic principles regarding pre- and post-operative management. There is no need for detailed knowledge on the procedure itself. Use this list to tick off the procedures when you feel confident of your knowledge.

GASTROINTESTINAL TRACT
- ❏ Oesophagectomy
- ❏ Billroth I and Billroth II (Polya) gastrectomy
- ❏ Small bowel resection
- ❏ Appendicectomy
- ❏ Hemicolectomy, subtotal colectomy, stomas
- ❏ Hartmann's procedure
- ❏ Anterior resection and abdomino-perineal resection of the rectum
- ❏ Haemorrhoidectomy
- ❏ Lateral sphincterotomy

VASCULAR
- ❏ Carotid endarterectomy
- ❏ Femoral–popliteal artery bypass graft
- ❏ High saphenous ligation and stripping of the long saphenous vein

BREAST
- ❏ Lumpectomy
- ❏ Mastectomy

THYROID
- ❏ Lobectomy, total thyroidectomy

UROLOGY
- ❏ Transurethral resection of the prostate (TURP)
- ❏ Nephrectomy

OTHERS
- ❏ Laparoscopic cholecystectomy
- ❏ Lichtenstein repair of inguinal hernias
- ❏ Nissen's fundoplication for hiatus hernia

ABBREVIATIONS

ACTH	Adrenocorticotrophin hormone
ADH	Antidiuretic hormone
AIDS	Acquired immunodeficiency syndrome
APTT	Activated partial thromboplastin time
AXR	Abdominal X-ray
CMV	Cytomegalovirus
CREST	Calcinosis, Raynaud's phenomenon, (o)esophageal dysfunction, sclerodactyly and telangiectasia
CT	Computer tomography
CVP	Central venous pressure
CXR	Chest X-ray
DNA	Deoxyribonucleic acid
DVT	Deep vein thrombosis
EBV	Epstein–Barr virus
ECG	Electrocardiogram
ERCP	Endoscopic retrograde cholangiopancreatography
ESR	Erythrocyte sedimentation rate
H^+	Hydrogen ion
HIV	Human immunodeficiency virus
HTLV	Human T-cell lymphotrophic virus
INR	International normalised ratio
IVU	Intravenous urogram
K^+	Potassium ion
MRI	Magnetic resonance imaging
Na^+	Sodium ion
NaCl	Sodium chloride
NGT	Nasogastric tube
NSAIDs	Non-steroidal anti-inflammatory drugs
PE	Pulmonary embolus
P_{CO_2}	Partial pressure of carbon dioxide
PTC	Percutaneous transhepatic cholangiogram
PVD	Peripheral vascular disease
RNA	Ribonucleic acid
RTA	Road traffic accident
TB	Tuberculosis
TPN	Total parenteral nutrition
USS	Ultrasound scan

NORMAL RANGES

Serum	Normal Range
Albumin	36–52 g/l
Amylase	70–300 IU/l
Bicarbonate	22–28 mmol/l
Bilirubin	5–20 µmol/l
Calcium	2.20–2.60 mmol/l
Chloride	95–105 mmol/l
Creatinine kinase	23–175 IU/l
Creatinine	60–120 µmol/l
Gamma-glutamyl transferase (GGT)	< 40 IU/l
Globulins	24–37 g/l
Immunoglobulins	
IgG	5.3–16.5 g/l
IgA	0.8–4.0 g/l
IgM	0.5–2.0 g/l
Iron	14–29 µmol/l
Iron binding capacity (TIBC)	45–75 µmol/l
Lactate dehydrogenase (LDH)	100–300 IU/l
Magnesium	0.70–1.00 mmol/l
Osmolarity	270–295 mosm/l
Phosphatase (acid)	0–4 IU/l
Phosphatase (alkaline)	40–115 IU/l
Phosphate	0.8–1.4 mmol/l
Potassium	3.5–5.0 mmol/l
Protein	62–82 g/l
Sodium	135–145 mmol/l
Thyroid function tests	
T_4	54–144 nmol/l
TSH	0.10–5.0 mU/l
T_3	0.8–2.7 nmol/l
FT_4	9–25 pmol/l
Thyroxine binding globulin	10–30 mg/l
Transaminase ALT	11–55 IU/l
Transaminase AST	13–42 IU/l
Transferrin	2–4 g/l
Urate	0.24–0.45 mmol/l
Urea	2.5–6.6 mmol/l

Normal Ranges

Plasma

Glucose	3.0–5.9 mmol/l
Arterial blood gases	
H^+	36–43 nmol/l
P_{CO_2}	4.6–6.0 kPa
Bicarbonate	20–28 mmol/l
P_{O_2}	10.5–13.5 kPa
Lactate	0.63–2.44 mmol/l
Pyruvate	34–80 μmol/l

Cerebrospinal Fluid (CSF)

Glucose	2.5–3.9 mmol/l
Protein	< 0.45 g/l

Urine

Catecholamines	< 1.3 μmol/24 h
VMA (HMMA)	9–36 μmol/24 h
5HIAA	10–50 μmol/24 h
Microalbumin	< 30 mg/l
Creatinine clearance	60–110 ml/min

Miscellaneous

Faecal fat	< 10 mmol/24 h
Xylose excretion test	
Urine excretion (25-g dose)	> 33 mmol/5 h
Urine excretion (5-g dose)	> 8 mmol/5 h
Blood xylose at 1 h (25-g dose)	2.0–4.8 mmol/l
Blood xylose at 2 h (25-g dose)	1.0–5.0 mmol/l

MULTIPLE CHOICE QUESTION PAPER 1

60 questions: time allowed 2½ hours.
Mark your answers with a tick (True) or a cross (False) in the box provided.
Leave the box blank for 'Don't know'. Do not look at the answers until you
have completed the whole question paper.

1.1 In the management of a patient with a head injury

- A the airway is not a problem
- B a raised blood pressure (eg 190/100) with tachycardia suggests hypovolaemia T
- C a patient who is groaning with their eyes open and who is localising pain has a Glasgow Coma Scale score of 11
- D a CT scan is mandatory F
- E a helmet should not be removed   F

1.2 Acute appendicitis

- A causes pain in the umbilical area which 'moves' to the right iliac fossa (RIF)   T
- B can be excluded if the white cell count and temperature are normal   F
- C can be mistaken for ovarian cyst rupture T
- D can be treated by laparoscopic appendicectomy   F
- E mimics mesenteric adenitis F in yey children

1.3 Carcinoma of the breast

- A is associated with Paget's disease of the nipple ✓
- B may be hormone-dependent ✓
- C should be treated by mastectomy
- D may be asymptomatic ✓
- E is detected by mammography on the NHS breast screening programme ✓

1.4 A chest drain

- A is essential for the treatment of pneumothorax
- B is inserted under general anaesthetic
- C is essential for the treatment of tension pneumothorax
- D is inserted for drainage of empyema
- E can be used to drain haemothorax

1

1.5   The carcinoid syndrome

❑ A   may include valvular lesions of the heart
❑ B   may be treated with antibiotics
☑ C   is characterised by flushing and diarrhoea
☑ D   can only occur with liver metastases
☑ E   may present as appendicitis

1.6   Osteoarthritis of the hip can be treated with

☑ A   total knee replacement
☑ B   steroids
☑ C   arthrodesis
❑ D   osteotomy
☑ E   hemiarthroplasty

1.7   Clinical features of hyperthyroidism include

☑ A   atrial fibrillation
☑ B   weight loss
❑ C   bradycardia
☑ D   intolerance to cold
❑ E   exophthalmos

1.8   Clinical features of prolapsed intervertebral disc at the L5/S1 level include

☑ A   back pain
☑ B   pain on straight leg raising
❑ C   absence of the knee jerk L3/L4
❑ D   loss of sensation on the outer border of the foot
☑ E   weakness of foot inversion

1.9   The carpal tunnel syndrome (CTS) is indicated by

☑ A   wasting of the thenar eminence
☑ B   Tinel's sign
❑ C   blanching of the fingers on exposure to cold CRESS / RAYNAUD
☑ D   paraesthesia of the thumb and index finger
☑ E   pain in the hand which is worse at night

1.10 With regard to obesity

- ☑ A open surgery is contraindicated
- ❏ B laparoscopic surgery is contraindicated
- ❏ C risk of morbidity and mortality is decreased
- ☑ D weight loss is essential before surgery
- ☑ E a body mass index greater than 28 is significant

1.11 The following refer to hiatus hernia

- ❏ A the treatment of choice is fundoplication ?
- ❏ B rolling hernias are more common than the sliding type
- ☑ C severe acid reflux occurs mainly in rolling hernias
- ❏ D it can be diagnosed by endoscopy
- ☑ E weight loss is advised

1.12 Perforated duodenal ulcer

- ❏ A may be treated conservatively
- ❏ B should be confirmed by gastroscopy before laparotomy
- ❏ C should be confirmed by CT before laparotomy
- ❏ D can present without abdominal signs
- ❏ E is excluded if the serum amylase is more than 500 IU/l

1.13 Duke's staging of colorectal carcinoma

- ❏ A involves assessment of lymph node spread
- ❏ B requires assessment of the depth of tumour penetration through the wall of the bowel
- ❏ C involves assessment of the presence or absence of metastases in distant organs
- ❏ D is made at post-mortem
- ❏ E requires measurement of the distances between the tumour and the resection lines

1.14 Ulcerative colitis

❏ A may be complicated by retinitis
❏ B should be investigated by rectal biopsy
❏ C may predispose to carcinoma of the large bowel, especially with early onset of total colitis
❏ D should be investigated by colonoscopy if there is dilatation of the large bowel on plain X-ray
❏ E is not commonly associated with protein loss

1.15 Common causes of small bowel obstruction in adults are

❏ A stricture due to rectal carcinoma
❏ B adhesions
❏ C Meckel's diverticulum
❏ D intussusception
❏ E strangulated hernia

1.16 Recognised consequences of achalasia of the cardia include

❏ A dysphagia
❏ B pneumonia
❏ C carcinoma of the oesophagus
❏ D absent gastric air bubble
❏ E heartburn

1.17 First-degree haemorrhoids are a cause of

❏ A rectal bleeding
❏ B anal pain
❏ C rectal mucosal prolapse
❏ D melaena
❏ E pruritis ani

1.18 Femoral hernia

❏ A frequently becomes strangulated
❏ B is more common in men than in women
❏ C causes swelling of the lower limb
❏ D may be confused with an enlarged lymph node
❏ E is more common than inguinal hernia

1.19 Endoscopic retrograde cholangiopancreatography (ERCP)

❑ A usually requires a general anaesthetic
❑ B is valuable for confirming a suspicion of acute pancreatitis
❑ C gives information equivalent to that obtained by percutaneous transhepatic cholangiography
❑ D is contraindicated in the presence of jaundice
❑ E can diagnose strictures of the pancreatic duct

1.20 Gallstones

❑ A are usually formed in the bile ducts
❑ B have been found in the stools
❑ C are causally related to carcinoma of the gallbladder
❑ D are usually radio-opaque
❑ E can cause acute pancreatitis

1.21 Typical biochemical features of serum in obstructive jaundice include

❑ A raised bilirubin
❑ B increased acid phosphatase
❑ C increased alkaline phosphatase
❑ D increased amylase
❑ E positive hepatitis B surface antigen

1.22 Splenectomy is likely to be of value in

❑ A congenital spherocytosis
❑ B myelofibrosis
❑ C malaria
❑ D infectious mononucleosis
❑ E agranulocytosis

1.23 A lump in the midline of the neck may be

❑ A a dermoid cyst
❑ B a sebaceous cyst
❑ C a thyroglossal cyst
❑ D a branchial cyst
❑ E a cystic hygroma

1.24   Carcinoma of the breast may present with

❏ A   *peau d'orange*
❏ B   shortness of breath
❏ C   lymphoedema of the arm
❏ D   a fracture of bone
❏ E   inversion of the nipple

1.25   In ureteric obstruction due to a calculus, an intravenous urogram would be expected to show

❏ A   normal excretion in the non-affected kidney
❏ B   delayed excretion in the affected kidney
❏ C   enlargement of the affected kidney
❏ D   contraction of the unaffected kidney
❏ E   the site of obstruction

1.26   A size 24 Fr catheter

❏ A   must always be inserted using aseptic technique
❏ B   is 24 mm in diameter
❏ C   is 24 mm in length
❏ D   is 24 mm in external circumference
❏ E   is the suitable first choice for urethral catheterisation of the adult male

1.27   Renal carcinoma in adults

❏ A   usually presents as painful haematuria
❏ B   commonly metastasises to bone
❏ C   may grow into the inferior vena cava
❏ D   may give rise to a cannonball metastasis
❏ E   is called a Wilms' tumour

1.28   A patient has a road traffic accident resulting in severe chest injury. He presents in severe respiratory distress and his trachea is deviated to the left. The first thing you should do is to

❏ A   request an urgent X-ray
❏ B   insert an exploratory needle into the second left intercostal space
❏ C   perform an emergency tracheostomy
❏ D   gain intravenous access
❏ E   obtain an electrocardiogram

1.29 A full-thickness burn of the right leg

- ❑ A is estimated to represent 5% of the entire body surface area
- ❑ B may cause a peptic ulcer
- ❑ C may result in thrombosis
- ❑ D is treated by resuscitation with intravenous fluids
- ❑ E should be covered with ice

1.30 Varicose veins

- ❑ A cause lipodermatosclerosis
- ❑ B should always be treated by injection sclerotherapy
- ❑ C are common in rural Africa
- ❑ D are more common in the short than in the long saphenous system
- ❑ E can cause serious haemorrhage

1.31 Intermittent claudication

- ❑ A is usually caused by atherosclerosis
- ❑ B is worse at night
- ❑ C may improve on continued exercise
- ❑ D may proceed to gangrene
- ❑ E requires surgery to the affected arteries

1.32 Clinical features of acute pancreatitis include

- ❑ A tetany
- ❑ B paralytic ileus
- ❑ C vomiting
- ❑ D jaundice
- ❑ E a pleural effusion

1.33 Symptoms of malignant change in a melanoma are

- ❑ A bleeding
- ❑ B hair in the lesion
- ❑ C change in colour
- ❑ D itching
- ❑ E satellite lesions

1.34   A fistula

❑   A   arises from a blind-ending abscess cavity
❑   B   will never heal spontaneously
❑   C   connects two separate epithelial surfaces
❑   D   may be found in the anal canal
❑   E   may give rise to severe fluid and electrolyte losses

1.35   Normal saline given intravenously

❑   A   is a solution containing one mole of sodium chloride per litre of water
❑   B   is a solution containing 0.9 g of sodium chloride per litre of water
❑   C   has the same osmotic pressure as plasma
❑   D   is a 0.9% solution of sodium chloride in water
❑   E   should never be given for hypovolaemia

1.36   In patients with chronic vomiting

❑   A   a metabolic acidosis results
❑   B   a metabolic alkalosis results
❑   C   there is excess loss of sodium in the urine
❑   D   potassium deficiency may occur
❑   E   there may be the same metabolic effect as continual nasogastric aspiration

1.37   Factors which favour wound healing include

❑   A   a good blood supply
❑   B   a haematoma
❑   C   tension
❑   D   the presence of bacteria
❑   E   a minimum of suture materials

1.38   Causes of hypotension in adults include

❑   A   an upper gastrointestinal bleed
❑   B   intracranial bleeding
❑   C   myocardial infarction
❑   D   infarction of the small bowel
❑   E   systemic infection with Gram-negative organisms

1.39   Nutritional problems seen after a partial gastrectomy include

- ❏   A   macrocytic anaemia
- ❏   B   osteoporosis
- ❏   C   weight loss
- ❏ `*` D   iron deficiency anaemia
- ❏   E   hypoglycaemia

1.40   Subphrenic abscesses

- ❏   A   are best treated by antibiotics
- ❏   B   occur after perforated peptic ulcer
- ❏   C   may be associated with a pleural effusion on the same side
- ❏   D   cause hiccoughs
- ❏   E   should not be treated by aspiration alone

1.41   The following are features of Horner's syndrome:

- ❏   A   dilatation of the ipsilateral pupil
- ❏   B   enophthalmos
- ❏   C   absent sweating on the affected side of the face
- ❏   D   deviation of the tongue to one side on protrusion
- ❏   E   ptosis of the ipsilateral eye

1.42   Clinical features typical of acute appendicitis include

- ❏   A   fetor oris
- ❏   B   fever
- ❏   C   pain in the right shoulder
- ❏   D   guarding in the left iliac fossa
- ❏   E   anorexia

1.43   In Bell's palsy

- ❏   A   patients may complain of impairment of taste
- ❏   B   there is unilateral facial weakness
- ❏   C   there is unilateral loss of sensation of the skin
- ❏   D   herpes zoster is the cause
- ❏   E   the voice is hoarse

1.44   Tearing of the medial meniscus of the knee leads to

- ❏ A   quadriceps wasting
- ❏ B   recurrent haemarthrosis
- ❏ C   limitation of knee flexion
- ❏ D   locking of the knee
- ❏ E   intermittent effusions

1.45   Avascular necrosis occurs in

- ❏ A   fracture through the waist of the scaphoid
- ❏ B   dislocation of the lunate bone
- ❏ C   subcapital fracture of the femoral neck
- ❏ D   steroid therapy
- ❏ E   caisson disease

1.46   Neuromuscular blocking agents that act by competitive inhibition include

- ❏ A   pethidine
- ❏ B   suxamethonium
- ❏ C   neostigmine
- ❏ D   hexamethonium
- ❏ E   tubocurarine

1.47   Carcinoma of the stomach is associated with

- ❏ A   blood group O
- ❏ B   cigarette smoking
- ❏ C   pernicious anaemia
- ❏ D   iron deficiency anaemia
- ❏ E   transcoelomic spread to the ovary

1.48   Minimally invasive surgery

- ❏ A   is used for cholecystectomy
- ❏ B   affords a quicker recovery than open procedures
- ❏ C   can be used for cervical sympathectomy
- ❏ D   is contraindicated in morbid obesity
- ❏ E   means minimal skill is required

1.49   A sarcoma

- ❏   A   is a malignant tumour
- ❏   B   spreads primarily via the bloodstream
- ❏   C   responds to radiotherapy
- ❏   D   grows rapidly
- ❏   E   has a good prognosis

1.50   Carcinoma of the prostate

- ❏   A   occurs frequently in men over the age of 65 years
- ❏   B   responds to testosterone therapy
- ❏   C   can cause a rectal stricture
- ❏   D   produces osteosclerotic secondary bone deposits
- ❏   E   spreads to pelvic lymph nodes

1.51   The following classically occur within 24 hours of an operation

- ❏   A   deep vein thrombosis
- ❏   B   pulmonary embolus
- ❏   C   pulmonary atelectasis
- ❏   D   wound dehiscence
- ❏   E   reactionary haemorrhage

1.52   Gas gangrene is treated with

- ❏   A   local applications of antiseptics
- ❏   B   benzylpenicillin
- ❏   C   adequate surgical excision of the wound
- ❏   D   primary suture of the wound
- ❏   E   blood transfusion

1.53   Benign breast change

- ❏   A   often produces cyclical pain
- ❏   B   is normally unilateral
- ❏   C   tends to progress in the post-menopausal years
- ❏   D   is pre-malignant
- ❏   E   produces diffuse lumpiness

1.54   Gynaecomastia occurs in

❑   A   carcinoma of the prostate
❑   B   chronic liver disease
❑   C   carcinoma of the breast
❑   D   peptic ulcer disease
❑   E   bronchial carcinoma

1.55   An abdominal aortic aneurysm

❑   A   may be seen on a plain abdominal X-ray
❑   B   may present with a collapsing pulse
❑   C   may be due to syphilis
❑   D   needs treatment only if it causes back pain
❑   E   usually involves the renal arteries

1.56   A nasogastric tube

❑   A   should be used to protect respiratory function in all patients with severe head injury
❑   B   should be spigotted and aspirated at regular intervals
❑   C   may be used for feeding
❑   D   is required in upper gastrointestinal bleeding to assess blood loss
❑   E   may be used in the treatment of large bowel obstruction

1.57   The following facts are true of pleomorphic adenomas and their treatment

❑   A   they occur in the parotid gland
❑   B   they are rapidly growing
❑   C   they can be safely removed by simple enucleation
❑   D   surgery may result in damage to the facial nerve
❑   E   surgery may result in Frey's syndrome

1.58   Which of the following conditions may predispose to the development of paralytic ileus

❑   A   laparotomy
❑   B   potassium deficiency
❑   C   lumbar sympathectomy
❑   D   fracture of lumbar vertebrae
❑   E   calcium deficiency

1.59   Carcinoma of the oesophagus

- [x] A   occurs most frequently in the middle third of the oesophagus
- [x] B   is predominantly squamous in type
- [ ] C   is a complication of oesophagitis
- [x] D   is associated with alcohol intake
- [x] E   occurs in Plummer–Vinson syndrome

1.60   **In acute cholecystitis**

- [ ] A   immediate cholecystectomy may be performed
- [ ] B   antibiotics are mandatory
- [ ] C   delayed cholecystectomy may be performed
- [ ] D   treatment includes laparoscopic cholecystectomy
- [ ] E   laparotomy is advisable

—————————— **END** ——————————

**Go over your answers until your time is up.
Correct answers and teaching notes are overleaf.**

MULTIPLE CHOICE QUESTION PAPER 1 – ANSWERS

The correct answer options for each question are given below.

1.1	C	1.31	A C D
1.2	A C D E	1.32	A B C D E
1.3	A B D E	1.33	A C D E
1.4	C D E	1.34	C D E
1.5	A C E	1.35	C D
1.6	C D	1.36	B D E
1.7	A B E	1.37	A E
1.8	A B D E	1.38	A C D E
1.9	A B D E	1.39	A C D E
1.10	E	1.40	B C D
1.11	D E	1.41	B C E
1.12	A D	1.42	A B E
1.13	A B	1.43	A B
1.14	B C	1.44	A B C D E
1.15	B E	1.45	A B C D E
1.16	A B C D E	1.46	E
1.17	A E	1.47	B C D E
1.18	A D	1.48	A B C
1.19	E	1.49	A B C D
1.20	B C E	1.50	A C D E
1.21	A C	1.51	C E
1.22	A B	1.52	B C
1.23	A B C	1.53	A E
1.24	A B C D E	1.54	B E
1.25	A B C E	1.55	A C
1.26	A	1.56	C E
1.27	B C D	1.57	A D E
1.28	None correct	1.58	A B D
1.29	B C D	1.59	A B D E
1.30	A E	1.60	A B C D

MCQ PAPER 1 – ANSWERS AND TEACHING NOTES

1.1   Management of a patient with a head injury   Answer: C

In the patient with a head injury, trauma management follows the standard ABC protocol: Airway, Breathing, Circulation. It is important to immobilise the neck during resuscitation. The response to hypovolaemia is tachycardia and hypotension. This is graded according to severity as follows:

	I < 15%	II 15–30%	III 30–40%	IV > 40%
Heart rate	< 100	Raised > 100	Raised > 120	Raised > 140
Blood pressure	Normal	Normal/Low	Low	Low
Respiratory rate	Normal	Normal/Raised	Raised 30–40	Raised > 40
Peripheral circulation	Normal	Cool, pale	Cool, pale	Cold, clammy 'SHOCK'

Hypertension and bradycardia suggest raised intracranial pressure. Pain can cause raised blood pressure and tachycardia, but careful neurological examination is necessary.

The Glasgow Coma Scale (GCS) score is calculated as follows:

Eye response:
1   No response
2   Open to pain
3   Open to command
4   Open spontaneously

Verbal:
1   No sounds
2   Incomprehensible sounds
3   Inappropriate words
4   Confused conversation
5   Orientated conversation

Motor response:
1   No response
2   Extension to pain (decerebrate)
3   Abnormal flexion to pain (decorticate)
4   Flexion withdrawal response to pain
5   Localises pain
6   Obeys commands

Investigations depend on the history and clinical examination findings. Loss of consciousness and retrograde amnesia suggest increased severity of injury. Neurological signs warrant a CT scan.

Exposure is necessary to make an accurate assessment of injury. A helmet should be removed, paying particular attention to neck immobilisation.

1.2   Acute appendicitis   Answers: A C D E

Pain often starts vaguely in the central abdomen (as the appendix is a mid-gut structure) and then localises to the right iliac fossa when the peritoneum becomes inflamed.

The absence of some of the typical symptoms and signs does not exclude a diagnosis of appendicitis. Symptoms include:
- right iliac fossa (RIF) pain
- nausea and vomiting
- loss of appetite.

Signs include:
- tachycardia
- flushed peripheries (especially the face)
- pyrexia – usually up to 37.5 °C
- fetor oris
- mildly raised white cell count.

The differential diagnosis for RIF pain is ovulation/ovarian cyst rupture or pelvic inflammatory disease. This is often difficult to differentiate and may require further investigations such as ultrasound or CT scan to assist in making the diagnosis.

In cases where the diagnosis is in doubt laparoscopy is particularly useful, proceeding to the definitive procedure. Laparoscopic appendicectomy is increasingly used.

In young children an upper respiratory tract infection may cause mesenteric adenitis which presents with pain in the RIF and can be easily mistaken for appendicitis. Other similar conditions are Meckel's diverticulitis, Crohn's ileitis and gastroenteritis.

1.3   Carcinoma of the breast   **Answers: A B D E**

Paget's disease of the nipple presents as a red, eczematous, bleeding lesion of the nipple. There is malignant change within the epithelium of the nipple, which shows 'Paget's cells' and there is associated intraduct carcinoma in 50% of cases.

Breast carcinoma may be hormone-dependent. The oestrogen receptor (ER) status forms the basis of endocrine treatment, eg with tamoxifen or anastrozole.

Breast-conserving surgery is now increasingly used, ie lumpectomy. Mastectomy is reserved for large tumours, central tumours or for patients who express a preference for mastectomy.

1.4   Chest drain   **Answers: C D E**

The treatment of pneumothorax includes the following:

- aspiration – in uncomplicated cases with < 20% pneumothorax this may suffice
- intercostal tube drainage
- pleurodesis is used in persistent recurrent cases.

A chest drain is commonly inserted using local anaesthetic. General anaesthetic is not essential. A small incision is made just above the rib. Blunt dissection is performed though the intercostal muscles and parietal pleura, using artery forceps. The end of the chest drain is then guided into the chest. The drain should be attached to an underwater seal and then secured in position. A chest X-ray is performed to confirm the position. The movement of fluid in the tube on breathing suggests correct placement.

It is essential to insert a chest drain **after** emergency relief of tension pneumothorax. Tension pneumothorax is treated with immediate insertion of a cannula in the second intercostal space in the mid-clavicular line. Following release of the air under tension, a formal chest drain must be inserted.

Empyema is found within the pleural cavity. It can be treated by 'closed tube drainage' or percutaneous drainage inserted under radiographic control.

Chest injuries may be associated with pneumothorax or haemothorax (or both).

1.5   The carcinoid syndrome   5HT   **Answers: A C E**

Carcinoid syndrome presents with:
- flushing
- diarrhoea
- abdominal pain
- bronchospasm
- pulmonary/tricuspid stenosis – late
- hepatomegaly.

Carcinoid tumours are found in the appendix, gastrointestinal tract and lungs. They may secrete 5-hydroxytryptamine (5HT) and other hormones. Symptoms are produced by excess 5HT which is normally metabolised in the liver; symptomatic patients tend to have metastases. Carcinoid of the appendix is usually incidental but can also metastasise to the liver. If the tumour obstructs the appendix it results in appendicitis.

Treatment of carcinoid tumour is by resection. Liver metastases can be embolised or treated with chemotherapy. Octreotide inhibits 5HT release and is used for symptomatic treatment.

1.6   Osteoarthritis of the hip   **Answers: C D**

Osteoarthritis is a degenerative condition of the joints ('wear and tear') with damage to articular cartilage. It occurs in the elderly, most commonly in the hips and knees or interphalangeal joints. Cartilage-wear damage is increased in load-bearing joints. Treatment consists of pain relief using analgesics and non-steroidal anti-inflammatory drugs. Steroids are not beneficial. Mobilisation and weight loss is helpful.

Surgery is indicated in progressive disease when movement is compromised. The joint destruction increases, causing worsening pain and producing deformity. The surgical options are:
- **arthrodesis** – the joint is fixed in a set position, resulting in a stiff joint, useful only when movement is not required
- **realignment osteotomy** – this is used in cases where part of the joint space is intact and weight-bearing surfaces are realigned
- **joint replacement with a prosthesis** – this is the treatment of choice in the elderly. Osteoarthritis of the hip requires total hip replacement, not 'knee' replacement – read the question carefully!

Hemiarthroplasty is used in fractures of the neck of the femur.

1.7   Clinical features of hyperthyroidism   Answers: A B E

The clinical features of thyroid disease are determined by examination of the thyroid gland itself and examination of all the systems for signs of altered thyroid status.

The thyroid gland itself may be normal or enlarged, with a single nodule or a multinodular goitre. It may have a bruit.

Hyperthyroidism causes:
- nervousness/anxiety/tremor
- increased appetite
- weight loss
- preference for cold weather
- palpitations.

Eye signs are:
- exophthalmos (Graves' disease)
- lid retraction
- lid lag
- dilated pupils
- ophthalmoplegia.

Hand signs are:
- tremor
- sweating
- acropachy (clubbing of fingers)
- onycholysis.

Cardiovascular system signs are:
- tachycardia
- rapid sleeping pulse rate
- heart failure
- atrial fibrillation.

1.8 Clinical features of prolapsed intervertebral disc at the L5/S1 level
Answers: A B D E

Acute prolapse of the intervertebral disc causes severe back pain with pain in the buttock and the back of the leg – sciatica. The clinical features are:

- muscle weakness and wasting
- reduced ankle reflex
- sensory loss on the outer leg and dorsum of the foot.

Herniation at L4/5 will compress the 5th nerve root and at L5/S1, the first sacral root.

L5 signs: weakness of knee flexion and big toe extension; increased knee jerk due to weak antagonists; sensory loss on the outer leg and dorsum of the foot.

S1 signs: weakness of plantar flexion and eversion of the foot; depressed ankle jerk; sensory loss on the lateral border of the foot.

Cauda equina compression causes urinary retention and sensory loss near the sacrum.

Acute disc prolapse may cause paraveterbral muscle spasm. Straight leg raising causes pain and is restricted.

Investigations include:
- X-ray
- CT scan
- MRI scan
- myelography.

Treatment includes:
- heat
- analgesia
- exercises
- rest
- reduction (bed rest and traction)
- removal of the disc prolapse by laminectomy or discectomy.

The patient will require rehabilitation.

1.9   The carpal tunnel syndrome (CTS)   **Answers: A B D E**

In CTS the median nerve which passes deep to the flexor retinaculum is compressed. Causes of CTS are:

- idiopathic
- pregnancy
- rheumatoid arthritis
- amyloid
- collagen disorders
- hypothyroidism
- oedema.

In the hand the median nerve supplies the muscles of the radial two lumbricals. It also carries sympathetic nerve fibres to the hand. It supplies flexor muscles of the forearm (except flexor carpi ulnaris and the ulnar half of flexor digitorum profundus). The features of CTS are:

- wasting of the thenar eminence
- pain in the hand which is classically worse at night, associated with burning and tingling
- loss of blanching of the lateral fingers on exposure to cold
- Tinel's sign – this consists of tingling in the hand produced by continuous tapping over the flexor retinaculum
- paraesthesia/numbness in the thumb and lateral two and a half fingers
- weakness of thumb abduction.

The median nerve roots are C6,7,8,T1. It passes lateral to the brachial artery in the upper arm and then crosses superficially at mid-humerus level to lie on the medial aspect of the brachial artery.

1.10   Obesity   **Answer: E**

Obesity is becoming significantly more common in the general population. The treatment of choice is conservative, ecouraging weight loss, diet improvement and exercise programmes. However, surgical treatment may be necessary and presents its own problems and complications. As always, these should be considered as 'early' and 'late' as well as 'general' and 'specific'. The complications are:

- **operative:**
  - general anaesthesia, eg difficulty with intubation, requiring 'rapid sequence induction', and difficult cannulation
  - drug metabolism is altered, requiring higher doses and intravenous access
  - surgery – technically difficult due to obscured access; takes longer

- **post-operative:**
  - DVT and PE risk is increased, especially due to slow mobilisation
  - wound infection
  - wound dehiscence
  - haematoma formation
- **medical** – there is a predisposition to:
  - cardiac disease, eg hypertension, ischaemic heart disease
  - respiratory disease – due to inadequate respiratory effort
  - diabetes
  - gallstones.

Surgery may be required to treat obesity (eg gastric stapling) or may be essential in obese patients who present in the emergency situation (eg strangulated hernia). Laparoscopic surgery can be performed in obese patients and this may be advantageous but requires skill and special long instruments for adequate access.

In elective cases, weight loss should be encouraged with the help of a dietician and a weight loss programme. A body mass index of greater than 28 increases the risks of surgery. Gross obesity doubles the risk of morbidity and mortality.

1.11   Hiatus hernia   **Answers: D E**

Hiatus hernia is classified into two types:

- **sliding** – 90% are of this type. The gastro-oesophageal junction (GOJ) slides upwards into the thorax, rendering it incompetent, and results in acid reflux and its complications (see Paper 2, Question 11). Management of any surgical case involves conservative measures, medical treatment and surgical intervention
  - conservative measures include weight reduction (to decrease the intra-abdominal pressure) and raising the head of the bed
  - medical treatment includes drugs such as H_2 antagonists or proton pump inhibitors
  - the surgical treatment is Nissen's fundoplication. There are variations on this procedure but essentially the GOJ is pulled back into the abdomen and the fundus of the stomach is wrapped around it

- **rolling** (para-oesophageal) – 10% are of this type, commoner in obese females. The fundus of the stomach rotates in front of the oesophagus and herniates through the oesophageal hiatus up into the mediastinum. Note that the oesophageal sphincter is not affected and so reflux is not usually a problem. This type of hernia can be asymptomatic but occasionally the stomach can strangulate.

1.12   Perforated duodenal ulcer   **Answers: A D**

Perforation is an important complication of duodenal ulceration. It may present without abdominal signs, particularly in the elderly and those on steroids. However, patients often present with peritonitis, the features of which are severe constant pain, rebound tenderness, guarding and rigidity, and absent bowel sounds. Other important features are tachycardia, hypotension and pyrexia. Abnormal investigations include leukocytosis, raised amylase (not as high as in pancreatitis), abnormal features on chest X-ray (gas under the diaphragm in 90%) and signs of free air on the abdominal X-ray (bowel gas shadows).

Management may be conservative, for example in the elderly or those unfit for surgery – symptomatic relief is provided while healing occurs as the omentum seals off the perforation. Surgery involves laparotomy with simple oversewing of the perforation.

1.13   Duke's staging of colorectal cancer   **Answers: A B**

Duke's staging of colorectal cancer is made by pathological assessment of the affected bowel and its local lymph nodes. It is therefore not an assessment of distant spread. It is as follows:
- **A**: growth limited to the wall of the colon (ie not through the serosa)
- **B**: extension through the wall and surrounding tissue but not to local lymph nodes
- **C**: metastases in the lymph nodes.

Stage D has been used to describe Distant metastases but this was not part of the original classification. In general, staging of carcinoma is useful to predict prognosis and further management, for example chemotherapy, radiotherapy, hormonal therapy, surgery. In colorectal carcinoma, surgery may be curative for stage A; for stages B and C chemotherapy may be added.

The five-year survival after operation is as follows:
    Duke's A – 95%
    Duke's B – 70%
    Duke's C – 40%

Note that 50% of patients with colorectal cancer are incurable at presentation and therefore do not undergo radical surgery with the aim of cure. These patients die within five years.

1.14   Ulcerative colitis   Answers: B C

Ulcerative colitis is an inflammatory disorder of the mucosa and submucosa of the large bowel. It is often complicated by systemic features. These include anaemia (of chronic disease or of iron deficiency due to rectal bleeding), seronegative arthropathy (20%), uveitis and iritis, skin lesions (eg, erythema nodosum and pyoderma gangrenosum) and, occasionally, sclerosing cholangitis.

Specific investigations include:
* full blood count for anaemia, urea and electrolytes, ESR as a measure of disease activity, rectal examination followed by proctoscopy and sigmoidoscopy with a biopsy if necessary
* abdominal X-ray may show colonic dilatation of toxic megacolon
* stool culture to exclude an infective cause
* contrast study – an urgent barium enema may be performed without bowel preparation, ie an 'instant enema', only if there is **no** toxic dilatation on a plain film. This may show loss of haustra, a lead-pipe colon, or filling defects due to pseudopolyps or carcinoma
* flexible colonoscopy – this is very useful to visualise bowel and permits excision of lesions such as polyps; it is used for surveillance. However, it carries the risk of perforation in fulminant cases of ulcerative colitis.

In young patients with total colitis for ten years the risk of developing carcinoma of the colon or rectum is about 10%.

Protein loss occurs as bowel mucosa is disrupted and sloughs off with blood.

1.15   Small bowel obstruction   Answers: B E

Please read the question carefully. It is advisable to know a list of causes but beware of the question that has been altered slightly. The answers can often be worked out logically. In stem 'A' the question refers to the small bowel and rectal carcinoma occurs in the large bowel!

Adhesions are a common cause of bowel obstruction. Meckel's diverticulum is associated with a congenital band which may cause small bowel obstruction but this is not common (the commonest complication of Meckel's diverticulum being inflammation).

Intussusception is when a segment of bowel becomes invaginated into the bowel distal to it, ie 'telescoping'. This answer is false as it is not **common** in adults, but it does commonly occur in children.

1.16 Achalasia   Answers: A B C D E

Achalasia is a disorder of oesophageal motility, resulting in contraction of the lower oesophageal sphincter. The proximal section becomes dilated. Patients are unable to tolerate either solids or fluids so that dysphagia is usually the presenting symptom. Fluids may spill over into the trachea, causing an aspiration pneumonia. Vomiting and retrosternal pain may occur in severe cases. A chest X-ray will show a widened mediastinum and possibly a fluid level in the oesophagus. A barium swallow shows a 'beak' appearance with dilatation of the oesophagus and a tapering constriction. The constriction prevents the passage of air into the stomach. There is an association between achalasia and oesophageal carcinoma.

1.17 First-degree haemorrhoids   Answers: A E

Haemorrhoids (piles) are abnormal dilated cushions of veins at the lower end of the anal mucosal columns. Symptoms of haemorrhoids include perianal irritation and itching (pruritus ani), pain, prolapse and bleeding. They are classified according to their position:
* first-degree haemorrhoids are not visible; they bleed after defecation and do not cause pain
* second-degree haemorrhoids prolapse after defecation, but then reduce spontaneously
* third-degree haemorrhoids prolapse and remain external
* fourth-degree haemorrhoids thrombose after prolapse.

Option C is false by definition. Haemorrhoids are usually located at the 3-, 7-, and 11-o'clock positions. They are situated above the dentate line and so can be injected painlessly.

Management is:
* **conservative** – high-fibre diet, avoidance of straining and good anal hygiene
* **medical** – local anaesthetic agents, steroids and symptomatic relief

- **surgical** – submucosal injection, banding, and anal dilatation are used for first- and second-degree haemorrhoids; haemorrhoidectomy is used for third- or fourth-degree haemorrhoids.

1.18   Femoral hernia   Answers: A D

A femoral hernia is the passage of peritoneum and its contents (including fat or bowel) into the femoral canal. It is quite likely to become obstructed or strangulated because the femoral canal/ring is narrow. The terms used vary but all have specific meanings, for example:

- irreducible – cannot be reduced
- obstructed – luminal contents obstructed but the bowel is viable
- strangulated – blood supply is cut off; leads to infarction.

Femoral hernias are more common in women than in men, but in both sexes femoral hernias are less common than inguinal hernias. A femoral hernia arises below and lateral to the pubic tubercle. It is usually small. If it enlarges it tends to be deflected upwards. A cough impulse may not be detectable and therefore it may be difficult to distinguish from a lipoma or an enlarged lymph node.

1.19   Endoscopic retrograde cholangiopancreatography (ERCP)
                                                          Answer: E

Investigation of the biliary tree includes:

- **abdominal X-ray (AXR)** – only 10% of gallstones are radio-opaque
- **ultrasound scan (USS)** – very useful to make the diagnosis of gallstones
- **ERCP** – used for imaging of the biliary tree and pancreatic ducts. It involves injection of contrast to outline the ducts. It allows the ampullary region of the pancreas to be inspected visually and the pancreatic duct may be outlined. It is helpful for identifying stones, strictures and tumours that cause obstruction as well as for therapeutic intervention, for example stone extraction or stent insertion where there is a blockage. Endoscopic sphincterotomy can be performed. It is particularly useful in the jaundiced patient and in those patients who are unfit for surgery
- **percutaneous transhepatic cholangiography (PTC)** – often used where ERCP fails, but it is more invasive. It involves entry via the skin into the liver and then injection of contrast into the duct system. There is no visual information of the pancreas. Stents can be placed via PTC but sphincterotomy cannot be performed
- **cholangiography** – this can be done operatively or via a T-tube.

1.20   Gallstones   Answers: B C E

Gallstones are almost always formed in the gallbladder (by precipitation from bile). They vary in content:

*   ~5% are pigment stones
*   ~20% are cholesterol stones
*   ~75% contain both.

Predisposing factors include high concentrations of bile, stasis and infection. Around 90% of stones are radiolucent. When a stone passes into the duodenum it may be found in the stool. Chronic inflammation of the gallbladder due to gallstones has been implicated in carcinoma of the gallbladder. Gallstones are present in most cases of gallbladder carcinoma. If a stone lodges in the ampulla of Vater it can cause acute pancreatitis. A stone lodged in the common bile duct can cause jaundice, ascending cholangitis or acute pancreatitis.

1.21   Obstructive jaundice   Answers: A C

In obstructive jaundice there is obstruction to bile drainage, preventing its normal flow into the duodenum. This is also known as 'extrahepatic' jaundice. As expected there is a rise in serum bilirubin and this is of the conjugated type as liver function is maintained. The urine appears dark as the excessive bilirubin is excreted by the kidney. The faeces are pale because of the lack of stercobilin which causes the brown coloration. (Note that urobilinogen is increased in the urine in liver cell damage and haemolytic anaemia. It is initially colourless in urine but darkens on standing.)

In obstructive jaundice, liver function tests must be performed. Typically they show:

*   bilirubin – raised
*   alkaline phosphatase – raised (liver isoenzyme)
*   transaminases – mild to moderate rise.

Acid phosphatase is raised in prostatic carcinoma. Amylase is a pancreatic enzyme which may or may not be raised in obstructive jaundice, depending on the cause of the obstruction. It is by no means typical. Hepatitis B causes infective hepatitis resulting in liver damage and intrahepatic jaundice.

MCQ Paper 1 – Answers and Teaching Notes

1.22   Spleen   Answers: A B

The spleen is a specialised lymphoid organ. It is highly vascular and is required for the maturation of white blood cells and for the destruction of effete red blood cells.

Splenectomy is indicated for:
- hypersplenism/splenomegaly
- staging of lymphoma
- excision of tumours, cysts or abscesses.

Splenectomy may be useful in the following conditions:
- autoimmune thrombocytosis
- autoimmune haemolysis
- portal hypertension
- splenic vein hypertension
- Gaucher's disease
- myelofibrosis
- trauma.

Splenic rupture is an indication for splenectomy. This may be due to rib injuries, blunt trauma or peri-operative injury. Certain infections, such as Epstein–Barr virus (EBV), malaria and infectious mononucleosis render the spleen susceptible to spontaneous rupture, but splenectomy will not alter the underlying disease as the question implies.

In agranulocytosis, white blood cells are deficient and hence splenectomy would be detrimental.

1.23   Neck lump   Answers: A B C

Dermoid cysts may arise from epithelium along lines of embryological development. They may arise in the midline of the head and neck and may contain hair or other ectodermal structures.

Sebaceous cysts are the most common skin cysts; they consist of stratified squamous lining epithelium filled with keratin. They are covered by normal epithelium and often have a punctum. They can occur anywhere but tend to occur where hair follicles are present.

A thyroglossal cyst occurs in the midline. It is situated anywhere along the midline, usually beneath the hyoid bone along the thyroglossal tract. This is the embryological tract of descent of the thyroid gland from the foramen caecum to its position in the neck. A diagnostic feature is that it moves on swallowing or protrusion of the tongue.

28

A branchial cyst arises from the remnants of the second pharyngeal pouch. It is typically a painless soft swelling, appearing deep to the sternomastoid muscle and bulging forward at the anterior border.

Cystic hygromas are lymphangiomas. They are present at birth and may be huge. They occur below the angle of the mandible on the side of the neck and not in the midline.

1.24   Carcinoma of the breast   **Answers: A B C D E**
Carcinoma of the breast may present with local symptoms, for example a lump, nipple discharge/inversion or skin changes, such as lymphoedema.

Paget's disease produces an eczematous change around the nipple. Locally advanced tumours may cause skin ulceration or even necrosis.

Axillary or supraclavicular lymphadenopathy may be presenting features. Lymphoedema of the arm may be caused by:
• surgery for breast cancer
• radiotherapy to the axilla for breast cancer
• axillary node disease.

Distant spread may occur to the:
• bone (sclerotic as well as lytic lesions)
• liver
• lungs (discrete metastases or lymphangitis)
• brain.

Bone metastases may cause fractures as a presenting symptom.

1.25   Intravenous urogram   **Answers: A B C E**
A ureteric calculus may cause obstruction to urine flow. The urinary tract proximal to the obstruction therefore becomes dilated and swollen. This is visualised on an intravenous urogram (IVU). For this procedure a 'control' abdominal film (KUB = kidney, ureter and bladder) is taken to look for opacities. Intravenous contrast medium is then injected and further film(s) obtained. Information is obtained about:
• renal size and shape
• speed of excretion of contrast
• the ureters
• filling defects/site of obstruction
• the bladder.

In acute obstruction there should be prompt excretion of urine by the unaffected kidney. The unaffected kidney should also be normal in size and shape.

1.26   Urinary catheters   Answer: A
A urinary catheter must always be inserted using aseptic techniques to prevent the introduction of infection. Usually a size 14 F or 16 Fr catheter is appropriate for catheterisation of the male urethra. The size ($\div 3$) indicates the diameter in mm.

Advice should be sought if there has been recent prostate surgery, if there is a urethral stricture, or if the patient has a history of difficult catheterisation.

1.27   Renal carcinoma   Answers: B C D
Renal carcinoma is more common in men than in women; the incidence increases after the age of 40. It is an adenocarcinoma and is also known as a hypernephroma because of its resemblance, under the microscope, to adrenal tissue.

Presenting features include:
*   haematuria, which is usually painless and may be macroscopic or microscopic
*   loin pain
*   abdominal mass
*   pyrexia of unknown origin
*   hypertension resulting from excess renin
*   polycythaemia resulting from excess erythropoietin
*   hypercalcaemia
*   secondaries, eg, cannonball metastases in the lung on chest X-ray or bone metastases
*   a left-sided varicocele – this is because the left testicular vein drains into the left renal vein, whereas the right testicular vein drains directly into the inferior vena cava; an obstruction to venous drainage by a left-sided tumour will cause back-pressure and hence varicosities of the left testicular vein, producing a left-sided varicocele.

1.28   Chest injury   Answer: None correct
In any case of trauma the primary survey consists of assessment of:
*   Airway
*   Breathing
*   Circulation.

It is important to remember protection of the cervical spine. The patient must be resuscitated to achieve stability of all the above. Following this, a secondary survey must be carried out to assess the patient from head to toe. This may be tailored to more specific areas suggested by the history and examination. The presenting features of a tension pneumothorax are severe shortness of breath and shock. The classic signs of a right-sided pneumothorax include decreased chest wall movement, tracheal deviation to the left, and hyper-resonance on the right with absent breath sounds. This is an emergency and requires immediate insertion of a cannula into the second intercostal space on the affected side. Following this, a chest X-ray may be obtained.

NB: You should not request a chest X-ray to diagnose a tension pneumothorax!

1.29   Burns   **Answers: B C D**

The estimation of the area of a burn is done by use of the 'rule of nines':

* head 9%
* arms 9% each
* back 18%
* front 18%
* legs 18% each
* palm 1%.

Major burns cause extensive fluid loss and this requires replacement with intravenous colloid and crystalloid. Hypovolaemia, together with haemoconcentration, predisposes to thrombosis. The insult to the body causes a stress response and peptic ulceration may result. Another consequence of a major burn is hypothermia, and ice would worsen this.

1.30   Varicose veins   **Answers: A E**

Varicose veins are dilated superficial veins of the legs. They are due to incompetence of the valves between the superficial and deep systems of venous drainage. The long saphenous system is involved in 90% of cases and the short saphenous system in 10%. Previous deep vein thrombosis predisposes to superficial vein congestion. Varicose veins are a disease of developed countries. Injection sclerotherapy is only of use in minor varicose veins.

Complications include pain (dull ache), cramps, ankle oedema, haemorrhage, thrombophlebitis, lipodermatosclerosis and ulceration.

1.31   Intermittent claudication   Answers: A C D

Intermittent claudication is characteristically described as pain in the lower limbs which occurs on exercise and is relieved by rest. The pain often occurs in the calf, but can also occur in the thigh or buttock. It is due to atherosclerosis. The outcome varies:

- one-third undergo spontaneous remission
- one-third can tolerate the symptoms
- one-third experience significant disability and restriction in their daily lives.

These patients go on to develop 'rest pain' and often hang their feet over the side of the bed to ease the pain (increasing the blood flow). If left untreated, they may develop necrosis or gangrene and require amputation. Some patients are able to 'walk through their pain'. This encourages the formation of collateral circulation and may help the symptoms.

1.32   Pancreatitis   Answers: A B C D E

Acute pancreatitis presents as an acute abdomen, with pain in the epigastrium or upper abdomen radiating to the back. It is worsened by movement and the patient can find no relief.

Vomiting is common.

Activated pancreatic enzymes are released into the pancreas, causing inflammation. Hypocalcaemia develops if there is extensive fat necrosis as calcium is then sequestered. This may result in tetany. A paralytic ileus develops and bowel sounds are often absent. Inflammation of the pancreas with oedema (or a mass in the head of the pancreas) may result in obstruction to the flow of bile and thus cause jaundice.

1.33   Malignant melanoma   Answers: A C D E

A change in the characteristics of a mole may be an indication of malignancy. Changes include:

- surface characteristics, eg increase in size, shape or thickness
- change in colour, eg darkening in patches
- itching
- bleeding
- brown halo appearance around the lesion
- satellite lesions – these are due to lateral spread around the lesion.

1.34   Fistula   **Answers: C D E**

A fistula is an abnormal connection between two epithelial surfaces. It is lined with granulation tissue but can become epithelialised. The fistula persists if the contents continue to flow along the tract, ie if there is distal obstruction to the normal outflow of the contents. If a fistula occurs between two loops of bowel (eg small bowel and colon) large amounts of fluid may be lost. A fistula in the anal canal is also known as a 'fistula-in-ano'. It connects the lumen of the anal canal with skin. Anal fistulae are classified into two main groups:

*   **low** – below the anorectal ring; this type is amenable to surgery by 'laying open' of the fistula, which then heals by secondary intention
*   **high** – above the anorectal ring; this is extremely difficult to treat because surgery may render the patient incontinent.

In contrast, a sinus is a blind-ending tract which connects a cavity with an epithelial surface.

1.35   Normal saline   **Answers: C D**

Normal saline is a solution containing 0.9% NaCl in water. This means there is 0.9 g of NaCl per 100 ml of water. Normal saline contains 154 mmol of sodium per litre; no potassium chloride is added. This concentration makes it isotonic with plasma.

A one molar solution of NaCl would contain 58.5 g (1 mole) of NaCl. In cases of hypovolaemia, intravenous colloid may be given as well as crystalloid to replace electrolytes.

1.36   Chronic vomiting   **Answers: B D E**

Patients with chronic vomiting tend to lose:
*   large volumes of water
*   hydrochloric acid (gastric acid in the stomach)
*   NaCl/K^+.

This results in metabolic alkalosis with a rise in pH. It is also known as hypochloraemic alkalosis. Continuous nasal gastric aspiration has the same effect. The patient becomes dehydrated and sodium is depleted. In the compensatory mechanism, the kidney acts to conserve Na^+ in exchange for K^+ and H^+. This is paradoxical aciduria because:
* H^+ is being lost despite the presence of an alkalosis
*   hypokalaemia occurs because K^+ is lost in the vomit
* K^+ is lost in the urine
*   alkalosis causes K^+ to enter the cells.

1.37   Wound healing
Answers: A E

Wound healing depends on:
- a good blood supply
- good apposition of tissues
- tension-free edges.

It is enhanced by a good nutritional state.
The detrimental factors are:
- infection – local or distant – bacterial proteolytic enzymes break down healing tissues
- foreign body, eg suture material
- devitalised tissue – due to poor blood supply
- haematoma – prevents good blood supply at the wound edges
- tension
- malnutrition – especially zinc and vitamin C deficiencies
- trauma
- metabolic diseases, eg diabetes mellitus
- drugs, eg cytotoxics and steroids.

1.38   Hypotension
Answers: A C D E

Hypotension is a sign of 'shock'. A common cause of this is hypovolaemia, eg as occurs in a gastrointestinal bleed.

Shock is due to underperfusion of tissues. It is often seen in infarction of the small bowel. Myocardial infarction affects the heart and its function. It may result in a significant decrease in cardiac output. Hypoperfusion results and blood pressure falls.

Gram-negative organisms, for example *Escherichia coli*, are well known for producing exotoxins. These act on the circulation and cause vasodilatation which results in hypotension.

Intracranial bleeding causes an increase in the intracranial pressure. The effect of this is to decrease heart rate and increase blood pressure (in contrast to hypovolaemia where the cardiovascular response is to increase heart rate and reduce blood pressure).

1.39 **Nutritional problems post-gastrectomy** **Answers: A C D E**

As with any operation, post-operative complications should be considered under the headings of 'early', 'intermediate' and 'late', with regard for the general and more specific complications of any particular operation.

Nutritional problems after a gastrectomy take several months to develop. They include:

- **dumping syndrome:**
    - as food passes rapidly through to the small bowel, the osmotic gradient draws water into the lumen. Hypovolaemia occurs and blood pressure falls; the patient becomes pale, cold and clammy
    - as carbohydrate-rich foods enter the small bowel rapidly, insulin secretion increases. When no further carbohydrate is present a rebound hypoglycaemia results
- **diarrhoea** – this is due to 'blind loop syndrome'. In the Polya type gastrectomy a blind-ending loop of duodenum harbours bacteria. Bacterial overgrowth then results in diarrhoea and malabsorption. Diarrhoea may be severe and episodic
- **vomiting** – due to overfilling of the stomach. Sometimes bilious vomiting occurs before a meal as bile refluxes into the stomach remnant
- **weight loss** – due to vomiting/diarrhoea and poor appetite (as there is no stomach there is no reservoir)
- **vitamin B_{12}** deficiency – loss of gastric intrinsic factor results in malabsorption of vitamin B_{12}. This causes a macrocytic megaloblastic anaemia. It takes between about three months to several years to develop as body stores are used up
- **iron deficiency anaemia** – normally the acid pH of the stomach increases iron absorption in the Fe^{3+} state. Therefore, reduced iron absorption results in iron deficiency anaemia
- **osteomalacia** – due to malabsorption of calcium and vitamin D. Also the acid pH of the stomach reduces calcium absorption
- **steatorrhoea** – this is due to poor mixing of food and enzymes, reduced pancreatic output and inactivation of enzymes in the afferent loops.

Other complications are:
- a feeling of fullness (the patient needs to eat small amounts of food frequently)
- gastric outlet obstruction
- ulceration in the gastric remnant (rare)
- tumour in the gastric remnant.

1.40   Subphrenic abscess   **Answers: B C D**

A subphrenic abscess occurs as a complication of intra-abdominal infection or surgery. The patient typically develops abdominal pain and a swinging pyrexia with sepsis where no other cause (eg chest or bladder infection) can be found. *E. coli* and *Bacteroides* are the most common offending organisms.

A subphrenic abscess can occur on the left or right side of the abdomen.

On the right side it occurs between the diaphragm and the liver. It communicates with the peritoneal cavity. Infection here commonly arises from the gallbladder or small bowel perforation.

Infection from the right kidney may also result in a right-sided subphrenic abscess.

On the left side it occurs between the diaphragm and left lobe of the liver, with the spleen further to the left. Infection is associated with gastric perforation or is from colon, pancreas or spleen.

Diaphragmatic irritation causes hiccoughs.

Investigations show:
* ESR – raised
* white cell count – raised
* CXR – pleural effusion occurs on the side of the abscess, empyema may occur
* ultrasound scan and CT scan – collections are visualised.

The treatment is:
* conservative, with antibiotics
* drainage – this is the definitive treatment; it can be by ultrasound or CT-guided.

Alternatively, surgery may be required.

1.41   Horner's syndrome   **Answers: B C E**

The features of Horner's syndrome are ptosis, miosis, anhidrosis and enophthalmos. Horner's syndrome is due to damage to the sympathetic nerves to the head and neck. The nerves involved are from T1 and its postganglionic connections, which synapse in the cervical ganglia. Interruption of the sympathetic nerve supply causes:

- the pupil to constrict
- blood vessels to dilate – vasodilatation
- reduced sweating
- drooping of levator palpebrae superioris: this muscle of the eyelid is supplied by sympathetic nerves as well as the 3rd cranial nerve. Interruption of sympathetic nerve function results in partial ptosis.

The causes of Horner's syndrome are:

- brachial plexus injury
- cervical sympathectomy – iatrogenic
- lung tumours, ie Pancoast tumour in the apex of the lung
- brain lesions
- syringomyelia or spinal cord lesions
- carotid artery aneurysm
- tumours in the neck.

1.42   Acute appendicitis   **Answers: A B E**

Acute appendicitis is a very common surgical emergency. The classic symptoms are as follows:

- pain – this starts as central abdominal pain which shifts to the right iliac fossa
- anorexia (before pain)
- nausea and vomiting
- constipation, but diarrhoea may occur.

The typical signs are:

- the patient is flushed, especially in children the tongue is furred, with fetor oris
- there is rebound tenderness and guarding in the right iliac fossa
- pyrexia (but the patient may be apyrexial) – if the temperature is greater than 38 °C consider perforation
- rectal examination may reveal tenderness in the right pelvic area.

The appendix is a vestigial organ attached to the caecum. Usually infection develops in the appendix because it is obstructed by a faecalith.

1.43   Bell's palsy   **Answers: A B**

Bell's palsy is a lower motor neurone lesion of the 7th cranial nerve, ie the facial nerve. The facial nerve supplies the muscles of facial expression, sensation to the external auditory meatus, and the salivary and lacrimal glands, and supplies a branch to stapedius. The features are:

- loss of facial expression on the affected side; there is drooping of the lip and lower eyelid. The patient is unable to smile, whistle or frown. On attempted closure of the eye, the eye tends to roll upwards. The lower eyelid droops and hence complete eye closure is not possible. The patient may require a protective eye patch and lubricant eye drops to keep the eye moist
- loss of lacrimation
- loss of taste in the anterior two-thirds of the tongue
- pain around the ear, due to inflammation
- hyperacusis if the nerve to stapedius is affected.

With a lower motor neurone lesion the entire side of the face is paralysed. In an upper motor neurone lesion the upper facial muscles are not affected because occipitofrontalis has a bilateral innervation and so when the patient is asked to raise the eyebrows they are still able to do so.

The cause of a Bell's palsy is unknown, although there may be a history of a previous viral illness. Treatment is conservative; the symptoms resolve with time. Steroids may be given, but their use is controversial. Around 40% of patients do not fully recover. A 7th nerve lesion associated with herpes zoster virus infection causing lesions in the external auditory meatus is known as the Ramsay Hunt syndrome.

1.44   Medial meniscus tear   **Answers: A B C D E**

Medial meniscus tears occur more frequently than lateral tears because the medial meniscus is attached to the capsule of the knee joint. This makes it less mobile and trauma is more likely to result in a tear.

If the cartilage then becomes jammed between the articular surfaces of the tibia and femur, 'locking' of the knee is felt, where full extension of the knee is not possible. Full flexion is still possible.

The patient may complain that the knee 'gives way'. The history is usually of a twisting injury resulting in pain and swelling due to recurrent effusions which may be haemarthrosis. In long-standing cases quadriceps wasting occurs. Investigations include arthroscopy or MRI.

Treatment:
- conservative – the leg is put in plaster with the knee extended for 3–4 weeks
- operative – this can be done at arthroscopy, eg suturing or partial meniscectomy.

1.45   Avascular necrosis   **Answers: A B C D E**
Avascular necrosis is ischaemic necrosis of bone. It is caused by interruption of the blood supply to the bone. It is a well-known complication of:
- trauma, such as fractures, eg of the scaphoid, femoral neck (subcapital), humeral head, lunate and talus, or dislocation, eg of the lunate bone
- caisson disease
- infection, eg tuberculosis
- neoplastic lesions
- metabolic, eg Gaucher's disease
- connective tissue disease
- drugs, eg high-dose steroids
- alcohol abuse
- vascular disease, eg sickle cell disease
- idiopathic, eg Perthes disease.

There is a useful mnemonic for remembering the causes of any condition – TIN MAN CAN DRIVE:

Trauma
Infection
Neoplasia
Metabolic
Autoimmune
Nutritional
Connective tissue
Ageing
Neurological
Drugs
Radiotherapy
Idiopathic
Vascular
Endocrine

1.46   Neuromuscular blockers   **Answer: E**

Muscle relaxants are often used during surgery. Neuromuscular blockers are of two types:

- **competitive inhibitors** (eg tubocurarine, pancuronium, atracuronium and vecuronium). These agents are reversible: they act by competing with acetylcholine for the receptor site. Remember that the neurotransmitter at the neuromuscular junction is acetylcholine acting on muscarinic receptors. Increasing the concentration of tubocurarine, for example, displaces acetylcholine and vice versa. Their action is terminated by the use of an anticholinesterase (eg neostigmine)

- **depolarising blockers** (eg suxamethonium). This agent is irreversible. Its initial action is to cause stimulation and hence muscle fasciculation may be seen. Patients often complain of muscular pain following an operation when suxamethonium has been administered. Suxamethonium has a rapid onset and is short-acting. It is normally metabolised by pseudocholinesterase. Note that some patients have a deficiency of this enzyme and in these cases the effects may be devastating. The deficiency is often familial and therefore a family history is very important.

1.47   Carcinoma of the stomach   **Answers: B C D E**

Carcinoma of the stomach is usually adenocarcinoma. The aetiology is unknown. The associations include:

- genetics – first-degree relatives have an increased incidence
- blood group A (duodenal ulcers occur more commonly in blood group O)
- geographical (eg the incidence is higher in Japan which is probably an environmental effect)
- social class – the incidence is higher in the lower social classes
- gastric mucosal atrophy predisposes to carcinoma (eg in gastritis and pernicious anaemia)
- polycyclic hydrocarbons and nitrosamines in the diet have been implicated
- cigarette smoking.

Carcinoma of the stomach is rare before the age of 50 years; it is more common in men than in women. Spread occurs locally, via the bloodstream and via the lymphatic system. Transcoelomic spread to the ovaries results in 'Krukenberg tumours'.

1.48   Minimally invasive surgery   **Answers: A B C**

Minimally invasive surgery refers to those procedures which are performed with minimal access, for example, laparoscopic surgery or ultrasound-guided abscess drainage. The incision is kept small. Laparoscopic surgery is commonly used for cholecystectomy and for hernia repair (keyhole surgery) but is also used for appendicectomy, fundoplication, hemicolectomy, sympathectomy and nephrectomy. The advantages are:

*   less operative trauma
*   a reduction in post-operative complications
*   quicker recovery time and restoration of mobility.

The disadvantages are that:

*   it takes longer (especially for inexperienced surgeons)
*   it is costly
*   exposure is limited
*   it has its own risks (for example, bowel injury during introduction of the Veres needle or increased risk of bile duct injury during laparoscopic cholecystectomy.

1.49   Sarcoma   **Answers: A B C D**

Sarcoma is a Greek word meaning 'fleshy growth'. It refers to a malignant tumour arising in the tissues of mesenchymal origin, for example, skeletal tissues. The suffix 'sarcoma' is used to denote malignancy. For example in bone the term used is 'osteosarcoma', in smooth muscle it is 'leiomyosarcoma'. Osteosarcoma occurs most commonly in the metaphyses of the femur. The cause is mostly unknown. However, there are several associations:

*   inherited conditions (eg neurofibromatosis)
*   ionising radiation
*   scars from thermal and acid burns
*   Kaposi's sarcoma, seen in AIDS.

Sarcomas tend to grow rapidly. Spread, as with any tumour, is:

*   local
*   via the bloodstream (this is the predominant route)
*   via lymphatics.

Note that in tumours such as those of the stomach, spread may occur via peritoneal fluids, ie transcoelomic spread.

Treatment of sarcomas is by a combination of surgery and radiotherapy. The use of adjuvant chemotherapy is controversial.

1.50   Prostate carcinoma   **Answers: A C D E**

Carcinoma of the prostate is the commonest malignant condition in men aged over 65 years. A patient may present with:

- no symptoms
- bladder outflow obstruction, ie hesitancy, poor stream, frequency, nocturia, post-micturition dribbling
- manifestations of spread (see below).

The modes of spread are:

- **local spread** – this involves local tissue, especially the rectum, and may cause a stricture: the patient complains of a change in bowel habit. Local spread may cause a major deep vein thrombosis of the lower limbs by obstructing venous return
- **distant spread** – via the bloodstream, especially to the pelvis and vertebrae; lesions are typically sclerotic. Patients present with bone pain or pathological fractures. The rate of growth depends on testosterone concentration.

Treatment:

- hormonal manipulation:
  - orchidectomy
  - oestrogen
  - luteinising hormone-releasing hormone
  - anti-androgens, such as cyproterone acetate (CPA)
- transurethral resection of the prostate – for early tumours
- radiotherapy.

When determining the pathology of a condition use the mnemonic,
In **A** **S**urgeon's **G**own **A** **P**hysician **M**ay **M**ake **S**ome **T**erribly **C**lever **P**rogress:

    Incidence
    Age
    Sex
    Geography
    Aetiology
    Predisposition
    Macroscopic features
    Microscopic features
    Spread
    Treatment
    Complications
    Prognosis

1.51   Post-operative complications   **Answers: C E**

Post-operative complications are best organised under the headings 'early', 'intermediate' and 'late':

- **early** – up to 24 hours:
  - atelectasis/respiratory distress
  - reactionary haemorrhage
  - urinary retention
- **intermediate** – second day to two weeks:
  - lungs – atelectasis, infection, pulmonary embolism
  - bladder – urinary retention, urinary tract infection
  - legs – deep vein thrombosis
  - wound – infection, dehiscence
- **late** – weeks later:
  - wound dehiscence
  - incisional hernia
  - recurrent condition.

These are general complications. Further consideration needs to be given to the complications associated with specific operations, for example, anastomotic leak in bowel surgery, nutritional complications following gastrectomy, or paralytic ileus and subphrenic abscesses following abdominal surgery.

1.52   Gas gangrene   **Answers: B C**

Gas gangrene develops when there is wound infection with *Clostridium perfringens*, a Gram-positive rod found in soil. It is an obligate anaerobe and therefore proliferates under anaerobic conditions. The organisms produce exotoxins which destroy tissue and result in necrosis. It produces gases which can be felt as 'crepitus'. Tissue destruction is rapid, initially blackening the skin which breaks down and becomes purulent. Necrosis occurs.

Treatment is:
- excision of necrotic tissue – the wound should be left open to allow drainage and **not** sutured; dressing packs are used to facilitate healing from inside out
- intravenous benzylpenicillin – should be given prophylactically in injury or before amputation of a limb
- hyperbaric oxygen therapy
- antitoxin administration.

1.53   Benign breast change   Answers: A E

Benign breast change is a benign disorder of the breast in which there is an abnormal response of tissue growth to the hormonal cycle. It may represent the extreme end of a normal range. It is not pre-cancerous but cancer may coexist and hence be misdiagnosed. Benign breast change (also called fibrocystic disease or painful nodularity) presents with:

- one or more areas of lumpiness
- cysts
- diffuse nodularity
- pain or tenderness.

These changes tend to occur in a cyclical fashion. The treatment is:

- reassurance
- lumpectomy
- mastectomy – very rare and only in severe debilitating cases.

1.54   Gynaecomastia   Answers: B E

Gynaecomastia is a benign condition in which there is enlargement of the male breast.

The causes are:

- physiological – neonatal or pubertal
- idiopathic – this is the most common non-physiological cause; it may be unilateral or bilateral
- chronic liver disease, eg alcoholism, cirrhosis
- hormones, eg oestrogens; in testicular atrophy hormonal abnormality may occur; hormone-producing tumours
- drugs, such as oestrogens – diethylstilbestrol (given in prostatic carcinoma), spironolactone, digoxin, cimetidine, steroids.

1.55   Abdominal aortic aneurysm   Answers: A C

An aneurysm is a localised dilatation of an artery involving all the layers of the wall. It may be fusiform or saccular. The most common cause is atherosclerosis.

Other causes include:

- congenital aneurysms
- trauma
- syphilis
- collagen diseases (eg Marfan's syndrome or Ehlers–Danlos syndrome).

2.5   Warfarin

- ☐ A   must be replaced by heparin before surgery
- ☐ B   may be reversed by protamine sulphate
- ☐ C   may be reversed by vitamin K
- ☐ D   is monitored by prothrombin time, reported as the international normalised ratio (INR)
- ☐ E   is mandatory after insertion of a prosthetic heart valve

.6   Deep vein thrombosis (DVT)

- A   usually results from incompetent superficial veins
- B   is prevented by heparin
- C   is treated with heparin
- D   is more common in malignancy
- E   is diagnosed by duplex scanning

7   Intussusception

- A   in infants usually requires resection of the bowel
- B   presents with bowel obstruction
- C   causes bleeding of the bowel
- D   is twisting of the bowel
- E   can be treated by barium enema

Splenectomy

- A   is indicated in congenital spherocytosis
- B   is of value in splenomegaly due to myelofibrosis
- C   should be preceded by *Haemophilus influenzae* immunisation
- D   may be complicated by gastric dilatation
- E   is followed by administration of long-term penicillin

Hoarseness of the voice

- A   is common in myxoedema
- B   may be a sign of anaplastic thyroid carcinoma
- C   may be a feature of laryngeal carcinoma
- D   usually occurs with pharyngeal pouch
- E   is severe in bilateral recurrent laryngeal nerve palsy

A genetic disposition has been found. The incidence is higher in men aged over 60 years; it is associated with hypertension and smoking. It may be asymptomatic or may produce a pulsatile mass in the abdomen, with abdominal pain radiating to the back. 'Shock' can develop if a leak or rupture occurs.

Aneurysms are most frequently found in the abdominal aorta and below. They are usually below the renal arteries. Calcification along the arterial wall often allows visualisation on a plain abdominal film. Other useful investigations are ultrasound scan, CT scan and aortography, which are used to assess size.

Size is monitored with serial ultrasound scans; elective surgery is indicated when the aortic diameter is greater than 5 cm, although this limit varies, depending on the fitness of the patient for surgery and the rate of expansion of the aneurysm. The risk of rupture increases with size and when symptoms occur. Surgery involves repair of the aneurysm with a prosthetic graft.

1.56   Nasogastric tube (NGT)   Answers: C E
In severe head injury where there is loss of the gag reflex, the airway needs to be protected. This can be done with a cuffed endotracheal tube. Insertion of a nasogastric tube is contraindicated in basal skull fractures as there is a risk of pushing the tube into the brain.

In small or large bowel obstruction the first line of treatment is 'drip and suck', ie intravenous fluid maintenance and suction of stomach contents via a nasogastric tube. The NGT is put on free drainage with aspiration at regular intervals. This relieves vomiting, protects the airway, and protects the dilated bowel from any further fluid and air. These conservative measures may be enough to relieve the obstruction. If not, surgery is required. Nasogastric aspiration is not useful in assessing upper gastrointestinal blood loss as a considerable amount of blood may be lost into the lumen and appear as melaena. A fine-bore NGT is used for enteral feeding.

1.57   Pleomorphic adenoma (mixed parotid tumour) Answers: A D E
Pleomorphic adenoma is an adenoma of salivary glands. Typically it presents as a painless slow-growing mass in the parotid gland. It is a benign tumour. The capsule is incomplete and the tumour may penetrate into surrounding tissue. It may then recur or undergo malignant transformation. Thus, enucleation is not enough for removal – excision is required.

At surgery, there is a risk of facial nerve damage as the facial nerve branches within the gland. Frey's syndrome occurs when the parasympathetic secretomotor nerve fibres to the gland are divided and then regenerate in the skin. This causes sweating on stimulation of the salivary gland, ie 'gustatory sweating'.

1.58   Paralytic ileus   Answers: A B D
Causes of paralytic ileus are as follows:
* laparotomy, ie handling of the bowel prolongs the ileus
* hypokalaemia
* peritonitis
* renal failure
* trauma (eg fracture of a lumbar vertebra)

Calcium is not implicated. Lumbar sympathectomy seems to prevent paralytic ileus.

1.59   Carcinoma of the oesophagus   Answers: A B D E
Most carcinomas of the oesophagus are squamous cell tumours occurring in the middle third of the oesophagus.

The risk factors are alcohol, smoking and diet (nitrosamines).

There is an association with structural abnormalities, for example achalasia, oesophageal webs, strictures, pharyngeal pouch and Barrett's oesophagus.

Plummer–Vinson syndrome consists of dysphagia (due to an oesophageal web) with iron deficiency anaemia and is associated with carcinoma of the oesophagus.

1.60   Acute cholecystitis – treatment   Answers: A B C D
Uncomplicated acute cholecystitis will resolve with [conservative treatment] ie bed rest, intravenous fluids, intravenous antibiotics and analgesia. Cholecystectomy may be performed early or late – about six weeks after the acute attack has settled. [Laparoscopic or an open technique may be used.]

MULTIPLE CHOICE QUESTION PAPER 2

60 questions: time allowed 2½ hours.
Mark your answers with a tick (True) or a cross (False) in the box prov
Leave the box blank for 'Don't know'. Do not look at the answers unt
have completed the whole question paper.

2.1   In the trauma situation, following an RTA

❑   A   screening X-rays should include cervical spine, chest and
❑   B   the treatment of a tension pneumothorax is immediate thoracostomy
❑   C   bleeding from a wound in the thigh should be treated by pressure on the wound
❑   D   open pneumothorax is treated with an occlusive dressing the wound
❑   E   pulse oximetry measures oxygen pressure

2.2   Avascular necrosis

❑   A   is a typical complication of fracture of the scaphoid bor
❑   B   is a typical complication of fracture of the femoral shaft
❑   C   may result from venous occlusion
❑   D   presents early with pain
❑   E   may result from arterial occlusion

2.3   The causes of an acutely painful swelling in the scrotu 11-year-old boy include

❑   A   epididymo-orchitis
❑   B   torsion of the testes
❑   C   hydrocele
❑   D   seminoma
❑   E   varicocele

2.4   A man sustains a laceration to the wrist from a brok dividing his radial artery. The following are appropr

❑   A   X-ray
❑   B   pressure dressing
❑   C   tourniquet
❑   D   tetanus prophylaxis
❑   E   nerve conduction studies to detect median nerve d

2.10   Which of the following statements are true

- ❏ A   diverticulosis coli results from a congenital malformation
- ❏ B   diverticular disease is pre-malignant
- ❏ C   diverticulosis causes rectal bleeding
- ❏ D   the diagnosis of diverticulitis is made on ultrasound scan of the abdomen
- ❏ E   pneumaturia may be caused by diverticulitis

2.11   The following occur with gastro-oesophageal reflux

- ❏ A   pneumonia
- ❏ B   oesophageal stricture
- ❏ C   iron deficiency anaemia
- ❏ D   polyneuritis
- ❏ E   pernicious anaemia

2.12   In gastric ulceration

- ❏ A   malignant change eventually supervenes
- ❏ B   an hour-glass stomach may occur
- ❏ C   excess acid secretion is the main cause
- ❏ D   carbenoxolone sodium may promote healing
- ❏ E   the majority of benign ulcers are situated in the greater curvature

2.13   Familial adenomatous polyposis

- ❏ A   may be inherited as an autosomal dominant condition
- ❏ B   is pre-malignant
- ❏ C   occurs in severe ulcerative colitis
- ❏ D   may cause electrolyte disturbance
- ❏ E   may be asymptomatic

2.14   Crohn's disease

- ❏ A   is familial
- ❏ B   is a malignant condition
- ❏ C   Reed–Sternberg cells are pathognomonic
- ❏ D   produces caseating granulomas
- ❏ E   is a transmural disease of the small bowel only

2.15   Symptoms of mesenteric embolus include

❏   A   rebound tenderness
❏   B   melaena
❏   C   hypotension
❏   D   visible peristalsis
❏   E   haematemesis

2.16   Constipation may be due to

❏   A   opiates
❏   B   aluminium hydroxide preparations
❏   C   hypothyroidism
❏   D   diabetes insipidus
❏   E   lactulose

2.17   Regarding haemorrhoids

❏   A   thrombosis is a recognised complication
❏   B   they can be treated with band ligation
❏   C   first-degree piles are best treated with haemorrhoidectomy
❏   D   they predispose to carcinoma
❏   E   strangulation can be treated with haemorrhoidectomy

2.18   Symptoms of a strangulated femoral hernia include

❏   A   irreducibility
❏   B   overlying redness
❏   C   tenderness
❏   D   diarrhoea
❏   E   a fluid thrill on coughing

2.19   Investigation of Crohn's disease often reveals

❏   A   a lead-pipe colon on barium enema
❏   B   increased uptake on a white cell scan
❏   C   rose-thorn ulcers
❏   D   strictures
❏   E   toxic megacolon

2.20   Recognised modes of presentation of gallstones include

❏   A   dysphagia
❏   B   abdominal pain
❏   C   shoulder tip pain
❏   D   small bowel obstruction
❏   E   tenesmus

2.21   Common signs of obstructive jaundice include

❏   A   dark stools
❏   B   dark urine
❏   C   splenomegaly
❏   D   itching
❏   E   a palpable gallbladder

2.22   Features of hydatid cysts in the liver include

❏   A   menorrhagia
❏   B   calcification on a plain abdominal X-ray
❏   C   haemoptysis
❏   D   anaphylaxis
❏   E   jaundice

2.23   A swelling presenting just below the angle of the mandible in a 30-year-old man may be

❏   A   a pharyngeal pouch
❏   B   an enlarged lymph node
❏   C   a thyroglossal cyst
❏   D   a carotid body tumour
❏   E   ectopic thyroid tissue

2.24   The incidence of breast cancer is higher in women who

❏   A   have already had breast cancer
❏   B   are young
❏   C   have breast-fed their children
❏   D   are obese
❏   E   have a family history of ovarian carcinoma

2.25   A hydrocele

❏ A   may be pre-malignant
❏ B   may occur after repair of a hernia
❏ C   occurs in the processus vaginalis
❏ D   causes infertility
❏ E   is reducible

2.26   A patient presents with a large swelling confined to the scrotum. It is transilluminable and the testis can be felt separately. The diagnosis may be

❏ A   a hydrocele
❏ B   an inguinal hernia
❏ C   a hydrocele of the cord
❏ D   an epididymal cyst
❏ E   epididymal tuberculosis

2.27   Acute renal failure following major abdominal surgery may be caused by

❏ A   hypotension during the operation
❏ B   a haemolytic transfusion reaction
❏ C   Gram-negative septicaemia
❏ D   blood loss
❏ E   fluid overload

2.28   After a head injury an extradural haematoma

❏ A   can be confidently excluded if the patient is conscious
❏ B   causes dilatation of the contralateral pupil at an early stage
❏ C   causes a deterioration in the level of consciousness
❏ D   is always associated with a fractured skull
❏ E   is characteristically associated with an increased heart rate and blood pressure

2.29   An undescended testis

❏ A   should be brought into the scrotum after the age of ten years
❏ B   is rarely associated with an inguinal hernia
❏ C   is prone to malignant change
❏ D   is more likely to undergo torsion than a normal testis
❏ E   means that the patient will be sterile

2.30   A varicocele

❏   A   may be treated by sclerotherapy
❏   B   is usually right-sided
❏   C   is associated with renal tumour
❏   D   can be treated by embolisation
❏   E   may cause pain

2.31   Raynaud's phenomenon may be secondary to

❏   A   carcinoma of the oesophagus
❏   B   pernicious anaemia
❏   C   atheroma of the subclavian artery
❏   D   carcinoma of the testis
❏   E   rheumatoid arthritis

2.32   Complications of acute pancreatitis include

❏   A   carcinoma of the pancreas
❏   B   stones in the common bile duct
❏   C   pseudocyst formation
❏   D   obstruction of the transverse colon
❏   E   fat embolus

2.33   Rodent ulcers

❏   A   are squamous cell carcinomas
❏   B   are basal cell carcinomas
❏   C   only occur on the face
❏   D   show epithelial pearls
❏   E   metastasise via the bloodstream

2.34   Recurrent anal fistulae are associated with

❏   A   Crohn's disease
❏   B   ulcerative colitis
❏   C   carcinoma
❏   D   Peutz–Jeghers syndrome
❏   E   diverticular disease

2.35 **A patient aged 65 years presents with severe abdominal pain radiating to the back, abdominal distension and hypotension. The likely diagnosis is**

❏ A   a leaking aortic aneurysm
❏ B   renal colic
❏ C   acute appendicitis
❏ D   acute pancreatitis
❏ E   pelvic inflammatory disease

2.36 **Tetany is a recognized complication of**

❏ A   metabolic alkalosis
❏ B   thyroidectomy
❏ C   a deep dirty wound of the foot
❏ D   overbreathing
❏ E   paralytic ileus

2.37 **An acutely infected ingrowing toenail may be treated by**

❏ A   Keller's osteotomy
❏ B   amputation of the toe
❏ C   lateral wedge excision of the nail and nail bed
❏ D   antibiotics
❏ E   nail avulsion

2.38 **In a man aged 50 years with a three-year history of indigestion, features of the management of one-litre haematemesis should be**

❏ A   a barium meal should be performed within 24 hours
❏ B   gastroscopy must be postponed for 48 hours after the last episode of bleeding
❏ C   in view of the history an operation should follow initial resuscitation
❏ D   blood transfusion should be started if the haemoglobin is less than 9 g/dl
❏ E   a careful watch should be kept on the pulse, blood pressure and central venous pressure

2.39 A pilonidal sinus is

- ❑ A a sinus containing hair
- ❑ B a fistula-in-ano containing hair
- ❑ C an abscess in a hair-bearing area
- ❑ D a sinus which commonly occurs in the natal cleft
- ❑ E often associated with a number of subcutaneous tracks

2.40 Malignant melanoma

- ❑ A is not always pigmented
- ❑ B may arise from junctional naevi
- ❑ C may itch
- ❑ D metastases in regional lymph nodes are very effectively treated by external radiotherapy
- ❑ E regresses after hypophysectomy

2.41 Buerger's disease or thrombophlebitis obliterans

- ❑ A affects young men
- ❑ B is confined to smokers
- ❑ C involves upper limb and lower limb arteries
- ❑ D is usually associated with Raynaud's phenomenon
- ❑ E affects the veins as well as the arteries

2.42 Carotid artery stenosis

- ❑ A may be asymptomatic
- ❑ B causes amaurosis fugax
- ❑ C causes vomiting
- ❑ D causes transient ischaemic attacks
- ❑ E is treated with carotid endarterectomy if the stenosis is 20%

2.43 In anal fissures the treatment is

- ❑ A laxatives
- ❑ B anal dilatation
- ❑ C examination under anaesthetic
- ❑ D often not required
- ❑ E excision of the fissure

2.44   Carpal tunnel syndrome may result in

☐ A   hypothenar wasting
☐ B   wasting of the interossei
☐ C   reduced sensation over the index finger
☐ D   a positive Tinel's sign
☐ E   pain in the forearm

2.45   In a compound fracture

☐ A   the bone is by definition broken into many fragments
☐ B   the overlying soft tissues are broken, with free communication to the exterior
☐ C   patients should be given appropriate antibiotic cover
☐ D   operative fixation of the fracture is contraindicated
☐ E   the bone is by definition broken in two or more places

2.46   Ranitidine

☐ A   acts by blocking histamine receptors
☐ B   is an H$_1$ antagonist
☐ C   is used to prevent stress ulcers
☐ D   can be given intravenously
☐ E   should be avoided in the first 12 hours following a gastrointestinal bleed

2.47   A peptic ulcer

☐ A   only occurs in the stomach
☐ B   may give rise to haemorrhage
☐ C   may cause obstruction in the duodenum
☐ D   is always associated with stress
☐ E   may be associated with hyperparathyroidism

2.48   The following are more likely to occur in ulcerative colitis than in Crohn's disease

☐ A   rectal bleeding
☐ B   abdominal mass
☐ C   steatorrhoea
☐ D   rectal involvement
☐ E   fistulae

2.49   Dupuytren's contracture is

❑   A   more common in men than in women
❑   B   associated with alcoholic cirrhosis of the liver
❑   C   associated with underlying malignancy
❑   D   transmitted as an autosomal recessive condition
❑   E   associated with renal failure

2.50   A closed fracture of the femoral shaft

❑   A   may be complicated by fat embolism
❑   B   may require blood transfusion
❑   C   requires tetanus immunisation
❑   D   may require intramedullary nailing
❑   E   will have healed fully within six weeks

2.51   Eighteen hours after an operation it is noticed that a patient has not passed urine. Which of the following would always be appropriate

❑   A   intravenous infusion of 10% mannitol
❑   B   injection of 20 mg furosemide (frusemide)
❑   C   catheterisation of the bladder
❑   D   examination of the bladder
❑   E   renal dose of dopamine

2.52   'Cellulitis' is a term used to describe

❑   A   death of liver cells in association with circulating toxins
❑   B   inflammation surrounding a malignant tumour
❑   C   spreading infection in the subcutaneous tissue
❑   D   tuberculosis involving the skin
❑   E   an abscess occurring in a surgical wound

2.53   Meckel's diverticulum

❑   A   is seen in 20% of the population
❑   B   is a remnant of the vitello-intestinal duct
❑   C   is a small appendix
❑   D   is associated with peptic ulceration
❑   E   may present as acute appendicitis

2.54 Salivary duct calculi

- ❑ A are more common in the parotid duct than in the submandibular duct
- ❑ B are usually radio-opaque
- ❑ C cause pain on eating
- ❑ D can be confirmed with sialography
- ❑ E are usually treated by surgical removal of the gland

2.55 Cancer of the stomach

- ❑ A has a five-year survival rate of more than 40%
- ❑ B is commonest in the antrum
- ❑ C metastasises to lymph nodes
- ❑ D may present with an abdominal mass
- ❑ E is treated by gastrectomy

2.56 Ureteric calculi

- ❑ A produce pain that is colicky in nature
- ❑ B should routinely be surgically removed
- ❑ C are predominantly 'triple phosphate'
- ❑ D can be treated by lithotripsy
- ❑ E predispose to transitional cell carcinoma of the ureter

2.57 The normal metabolic response to trauma is characterised by

- ❑ A an increase in lean body mass
- ❑ B antidiuretic hormone release
- ❑ C gluconeogenesis
- ❑ D a positive nitrogen balance
- ❑ E potassium loss

2.58 The passage of bright red blood with faeces may be caused by

- ❑ A a thrombosed haemorrhoid
- ❑ B anal fissure
- ❑ C ischiorectal abscess
- ❑ D carcinoma of the colon at the hepatic flexure
- ❑ E haemorrhoids

2.59   Staging of breast tumours

❏   A   assesses extent of spread
❏   B   indicates prognosis
❏   C   does not take account of nodal involvement
❏   D   is performed by mammography
❏   E   is only of use in women

2.60   Hypocalcaemia may occur in

❏   A   multiple myeloma
❏   B   parathyroid adenoma
❏   C   acute pancreatitis
❏   D   gallstones
❏   E   post-thyroidectomy

───────────────   **END**   ───────────────

Go over your answers until your time is up.
Correct answers and teaching notes are overleaf.

MULTIPLE CHOICE QUESTION PAPER 2 – ANSWERS

The correct answer options for each question are given below.

2.1	A C D	2.31	C E
2.2	A C E	2.32	C E
2.3	A B	2.33	B
2.4	A B D	2.34	A B C
2.5	C D E	2.35	A D
2.6	B C D E	2.36	A B D
2.7	B C E	2.37	C D E
2.8	A B C D E	2.38	D E
2.9	B C	2.39	A D E
2.10	E	2.40	A B C
2.11	A B C	2.41	A B C E
2.12	B D	2.42	A B D
2.13	A B D E	2.43	A B D
2.14	None correct	2.44	C D E
2.15	A B C	2.45	B C
2.16	A B C	2.46	A C D
2.17	A B E	2.47	B C E
2.18	A B C	2.48	A D
2.19	B C D	2.49	A B
2.20	B C D	2.50	A B D
2.21	B D E	2.51	C D
2.22	B C D E	2.52	C
2.23	B D	2.53	B D E
2.24	A D E	2.54	B C D
2.25	B C	2.55	B C D E
2.26	C D	2.56	A D
2.27	A B C D	2.57	B C E
2.28	C	2.58	B E
2.29	C D	2.59	A B
2.30	C D E	2.60	C E

MCQ PAPER 2 – ANSWERS AND TEACHING NOTES

2.1   In the trauma situation, following an RTA   Answers: A C D
The important screening X-rays in the trauma patient are the cervical spine, chest and pelvis. Further X-rays are directed at areas of interest.

Tension pneumothorax is treated by the insertion of a cannula into the second intercostal space (below the second rib), mid-clavicular line, for immediate release of air. The definitive procedure would then be chest drain insertion.

Bleeding is best controlled by direct pressure if the source is obvious and amenable. In open pneumothorax, an occlusive dressing prevents air being 'sucked' into the chest and expanding the pneumothorax.

Pulse oximetry measures percentage saturation of oxygen in the blood, ie SaO_2 percentage. Arterial blood gas measurements are used to determine PaO_2 = partial pressure of oxygen in the arteries.

2.2   Avascular necrosis   Answers: A C E
Avascular necrosis of bone is due to impaired blood supply, resulting in ischaemic damage to the bone. The causes are:
*   trauma – damaged arterial supply or venous occlusion
*   infection
*   vasculitis
*   sickle cell disease
*   high-dose steroids.

Certain fractures are particularly susceptible to ischaemic necrosis, eg:
*   femoral head and condyles
*   head of humerus
*   scaphoid, lunate, talus.

These rely on a main nutrient artery and have little collateral circulation.

Clinical features: the early stage is asymptomatic. Pain is usually the presenting symptom but occurs late when bone damage has occurred.

2.3 Causes of an acutely painful swelling in the scrotum of an 11-year-old boy   Answers: A B

There are two important descriptive words in this question. Firstly, 'acute' and, secondly, 'painful'. There are usually few questions on paediatric surgery but it is essential to know the important emergency conditions.

Torsion of the testes requires prompt emergency surgery before ischaemic damage results in necrosis, requiring orchidectomy. It is classically seen in children or adolescents presenting with severe pain of the scrotum, of sudden onset. There may be a history of mild trauma and/or previous episodes of pain. Examination reveals swelling of the scrotum with oedema and a horizontally placed testis. The scrotum is usually exquisitely painful, making palpation of the testicular artery very difficult. The differential diagnosis is epididymo-orchitis. This is a common condition, requiring analgesia and antibiotics; the onset is less acute.

Other causes include:
* trauma
* torsion of a testicular appendage
* strangulated inguinal hernia.

Seminoma occurs between 30 and 40 years of age whereas teratoma occurs in a younger age group, 20–30 years.

Varicocele is varicosities of the veins of the pampiniform plexus. It causes swelling which may disappear on lying down. It is not painful unless thrombosis occurs.

2.4 A man sustains a laceration to the wrist from broken glass, dividing his radial artery   Answers: A B D

The initial treatment involves management of the airway, breathing and circulation (ABC). Haemorrhage is best stopped in the acute phase by compression at the point of bleeding. A tourniquet is dangerous as it compromises the remaining circulation.

X-rays are useful for detecting glass fragments although not infallible. Tetanus prophylaxis is mandatory tetanus immunoglobulin and should be given if there has been no previous vaccination.

The median nerve may be damaged and the signs will suggest this. Nerve conduction studies are helpful after the acute injury.

Clinical features include:
- **motor function** – loss of abduction of the thumb. Later, the thenar eminence becomes wasted
- **sensory loss** over the palmar aspect of the thumb and lateral two and a half fingers.

2.5   Warfarin   Answers: C D E

Warfarin is an anticoumarin. It is a vitamin K analogue and reduces the vitamin K clotting factors. Its effects are measured by prothrombin time, represented as the INR.

Anticoagulation is often reduced before surgery to an INR of 1.5. If there is a high risk of bleeding, warfarin is withheld for three days before surgery to reduce its effects and substituted with heparin which is more controllable. Heparin has a shorter half-life and can be reversed quickly by protamine sulphate.

Patients on warfarin for atrial fibrillation need only omit their dosage and resume after operation.

Patients with prosthetic heart valves, where the risk of thrombosis is high, require continuous anticoagulation. Patients with prosthetic heart valves are maintained on permanent oral warfarin anticoagulation. Patients with tissue (porcine) valves do not require anticoagulants.

2.6   Deep vein thrombosis (DVT)   Answers: B C D E

DVT is a post-operative complication. There is an increased risk in:
- the elderly
- immobile patients
- malignancy
- abdominal and pelvic surgery
- orthopaedic surgery
- pro-thrombotic blood disorders, eg protein C deficiency, protein S deficiency, antithrombin III deficiency and factor V Leiden.

Superficial vein incompetence may be a contributing factor but is not usually the cause.

Investigations include duplex scanning and venography. Duplex scanning is unreliable below the knee. A blood test for D-dimers is helpful but has a high false positive rate.

DVT prophylaxis is essential. It should include:
* early mobilisation following surgery
* intermittent pneumatic compression peri-operatively
* compression stockings
* subcutaneous heparin or fractionated low molecular weight heparin
* avoidance of hormonal preparations.

Aspirin has antiplatelet action and will reduce thrombosis. Treatment involves anticoagulation with intravenous heparin, compression stockings and then conversion to oral anticoagulation with warfarin.

2.7 Intussusception
Answers: B C E

Intussusception is the prolapse of the bowel into itself causing a telescopic effect. It affects the ileum and/or colon, ileo-colic being the most common. There may be a focus such as a polyp or carcinoma which forms the apex of the intussusception.

Most occur in infants, in whom viral infection causes lymphadenopathy and this may propagate the intussusception. Bowel obstruction may result. Vomiting occurs.

The blood supply to the bowel is compromised. Bleeding may occur – this causes the appearance of what is described as 'redcurrant jelly' on rectal examination. Gangrene of the bowel and peritonitis ensues.

'Twisting' of the bowel is 'volvulus'.

Investigation of intussusception is by barium enema which is diagnostic as well as therapeutic, the weight of the barium reducing the intussusception. Otherwise, laparotomy is required for minimal reduction of the intussusception or resection of the ischaemic bowel.

2.8 Splenectomy
Answers: A B C D E

Splenomegaly is caused by:
* haematological disease, eg leukaemia, lymphoma, myelofibrosis, polycythaemia rubra vera, spherocytosis, β-thalassemia
* infections, eg glandular fever, typhoid, typhus, malaria, schistosomiasis
* Gaucher's disease, amyloid, collagen disease, sepsis
* cysts, tumours

- portal hypertension.

Massive splenomegaly is an indication for splenectomy. Other indications are:
- rupture following trauma
- uncontrolled splenic bleeding during colonic surgery (iatrogenic).

The complications of splenectomy are:
- gastric dilatation requiring a nasogastric tube and aspiration
- thrombocytosis immediately post-operatively. There is a risk of deep vein thrombosis – aspirin should be given
- sepsis. The spleen clears encapsulated micro-organisms, eg pneumococcus (→ pneumovax), meningococcus (→ meningovax), *Haemophilus influenzae* (give Hib vaccine).

Patients should therefore be given prophylactic vaccination pre-operatively. After splenectomy low-dose penicillin is administered daily to prevent overwhelming infection.

In splenectomy for trauma, pre-operative vaccination is not possible and the vaccine should be administered one week after splenectomy.

2.9 Hoarseness of the voice   Answers: B C

Myxoedema is hypothyroidism. It usually affects women over the age of 50 years. The voice becomes deep and slow. Other features are:
- bradycardia
- constipation
- thick, coarse, dry skin
- thin hair.

In thyroid disease the vocal chords are affected when there is infiltration of the recurrent laryngeal nerves. This occurs in thyroid carcinoma, especially anaplastic thyroid carcinoma. Laryngoscopy to check the vocal chords should be performed routinely in all patients before thyroid surgery.

Bilateral recurrent laryngeal nerve palsy will cause loss of voice. Both vocal chords are then held in the neutral position and this causes respiratory difficulty.

The recurrent laryngeal nerve supplies all the intrinsic laryngeal muscles except for the cricothyroid which is supplied by the superior laryngeal nerve.

Laryngeal carcinoma may of course affect the voice directly. The left recurrent laryngeal nerve may be affected in bronchial or oesophageal carcinoma.

Pharyngeal pouch causes dysphagia. The pouch arises at the junction of the pharynx and the oesophagus and consists of a mucosal outpouching between the inferior constrictor muscle and the cricopharyngeal muscle (Killian's dehiscence). Regurgitation of food may occur with aspiration but the voice is not usually affected.

2.10 Diverticular disease **Answer: E**

Diverticulosis coli is an acquired condition. It is due to mucosa herniating through weak areas of muscle in the large bowel wall, following high intraluminal pressures from peristalsis. The sigmoid colon is the most commonly affected part but diverticula may be present in any part of the colon.

Diverticulosis refers to the asymptomatic condition.

Inflammation of a diverticulum (or several) is called 'diverticulitis' which is then symptomatic. The common symptoms are:

- left iliac fossa pain
- fever
- rectal bleeding.

This leads to complications such as abscess formation, perforation, obstruction, adhesion formation, colovesical fistula formation and stricture formation. A colovesical fistula presents with pneumaturia and cystitis.

Diverticular disease is not pre-malignant. Diagnosis of diverticular disease is best made on barium enema or colonoscopy. Ultrasound scan is useful to detect abscess formation.

Barium enema or colonoscopy is performed after the episode of acute inflammation has resolved to reduce the risk of perforation.

2.11 Gastro-oesophageal reflux **Answers: A B C**

Reflux of acid from the stomach into the oesophagus causes oesophagitis. This presents with retrosternal pain, regurgitation and dyspepsia. Bleeding may occur, resulting in iron deficiency anaemia. In chronic oesophagitis, fibrosis occurs which may result in stricture formation and then presents as

dysphagia. Metaplasia of oesophageal epithelium from squamous to columnar may occur. This is known as Barrett's oesophagus, which is pre-malignant. Pernicious anaemia is associated with atrophic gastritis, not oesophagitis.

Reflux may be so marked that it causes overspill into the trachea. This is particularly marked at night when the patient lies flat, causing 'nocturnal asthma'; pneumonitis may occur. Other modes of presentation are halitosis and hoarseness of the voice.

2.12   Gastric ulcers   Answers: B D
Most gastric ulcers occur on the lesser curve. Frequency increases with age and there is an association with blood group A. It is more common in lower socio-economic classes. Acid secretion tends to be normal or low. The main problem is thought to be reduced mucosal resistance to acid (in contrast to duodenal ulcers where acid secretion is abnormally high).

Cigarette smoking is another association.

Helicobacter pylori is associated with both gastric and duodenal ulcers and therefore eradication therapy plays an important role.

Weight loss is a significant symptom in gastric ulceration as eating often causes pain, whereas in duodenal ulceration pain is relieved by food.

Gastric ulceration may be benign or malignant. Whether benign ulcers progress to malignancy remains controversial.

2.13   Familial adenomatous polyposis   Answers: A B D E
Familial adenomatous polyposis (FAP) is an autosomal dominant inherited condition. It is characterised by multiple polyps throughout the colon and rectum. It develops in teenage years when it is initially asymptomatic and benign. Later, symptoms develop and patients present with a change in bowel habit, eg loose stools, rectal bleeding and mucus per rectum. Malignant change inevitably occurs within 20 years. Prophylactic surgery is the treatment of choice, with total colectomy and ileorectal anastomosis or pouch-anal anastomosis. In ulcerative colitis, inflammatory polyps may occur, but this is not the inherited condition FAP. Electrolyte disturbance occurs when there is considerable loss of mucus and blood per rectum.

2.14   Crohn's disease   **Answer: None correct**

The aetiology of Crohn's disease is unknown. There may be a genetic predisposition as there is an association with family history.

Pathology: Crohn's disease can occur anywhere along the gastrointestinal tract from the mouth to the anus. It is characterised by:
- transmural involvement of the bowel, ie it affects the whole thickness of the wall
- granuloma formation (non-caseating)
- skip lesions, ie patchy involvement with normal areas in between
- inflammation and oedema of the bowel wall
- deep ulceration.

It is not a malignant condition.

Reed–Sternberg cells are seen in Hodgkin's disease.

2.15   Mesenteric embolus   **Answers: A B C**

Mesenteric ischaemia is a lack of blood supply to the mesentery. This may be due to:
- embolus
- thrombosis
- reduced cardiac output (eg due to myocardial infarction)
- blocked venous drainage
- hypovolaemia.

In mesenteric embolus, oedema of the bowel wall may result in rupture of blood vessels, resulting in haemorrhage into the bowel. The signs are:
- abdominal pain with rebound tenderness
- pyrexia
- dehydration
- vomiting
- white cell count > 30, 000/mm^3
- acidosis.

Abdominal signs are often mild and deceptive, even with extensive bowel damage.

The signs of generalised peritonitis occur if there is perforation. Some 90% of mesenteric emboli arise from the heart in association with atrial fibrillation. The extent of bowel affected depends on the site of final impaction.

2.16   Constipation   **Answers: A B C**

The causes of constipation are:
- drugs (eg opiates, iron, aluminium hydroxide preparations)
- hypothyroidism
- inactivity
- low-fibre diet
- faecal impaction
- bowel strictures (eg in diverticular disease or carcinoma).

'Absolute constipation' refers to the absence of flatus and faeces.

2.17   Haemorrhoids   **Answers: A B E**

See also the explanation to Paper 1, Question 17.

The management of haemorrhoids is as follows:
- conservative – high-fibre diet, avoidance of straining, and good anal hygiene
- medical – local anaesthetic agents, steroids and symptomatic relief
- surgical – submucosal injection, banding, and anal dilatation are used for first- and second-degree haemorrhoids; haemorrhoidectomy is used for third- or fourth-degree haemorrhoids.

2.18   Femoral hernia   **Answers: A B C**

See also Paper 1, Question 18.

A strangulated femoral hernia typically presents as an irreducible lump in the groin, with pain and tenderness. Overlying redness occurs due to local inflammation, especially in obstruction. If there is obstruction then vomiting, abdominal distension and constipation occur.

A fluid thrill on coughing suggests a saphena varix.

2.19   Crohn's disease – X-ray features   **Answers: B C D**

Crohn's disease is investigated with contrast studies:
- small bowel – a small bowel barium meal and follow-through or small bowel enema
- large bowel – barium enema.

X-rays show:
- terminal ileum – irregularity of the mucosa
- rose-thorn ulcers
- cobblestone appearance of the mucosa

- narrowing where there is fibrosis producing strictures
- dilatation of the bowel proximal to strictures
- fistulae.

White cell scans are performed to localise sites of inflammation.

Colonoscopy is often helpful to obtain biopsies.

The 'lead-pipe colon' is a feature of ulcerative colitis where there is loss of haustra.

Toxic megacolon is a feature of ulcerative colitis.

2.20 Gallstones   Answers: B C D

The modes of presentation of gallstones are:
- asymptomatic, ie an incidental finding
- acute cholecystitis – this occurs when a stone in the cystic duct or bile duct causes inflammation and transient obstruction
- chronic cholecystitis
- biliary colic due to attempts to pass the stone
- acute pancreatitis when stones impact in the ampulla of Vater
- obstructive jaundice
- small bowel obstruction due to 'gallstone ileus'; stones may impact in the terminal ileum
- empyema – a pus-filled gallbladder following stone impaction causes a swinging pyrexia and systemic illness
- perforation of the gallbladder producing peritonitis
- referred pain to the right shoulder.

2.21 Obstructive jaundice   Answers: B D E

The features of obstructive jaundice are:
- icterus
- pain
- malaise
- loss of appetite
- pale stools and dark urine.

A raised bilirubin causes yellow discoloration of the skin and sclera. If a clotting disturbance occurs, bruising may be a feature.

Courvoisier's law states that in the presence of a painless and palpable gallbladder, jaundice is unlikely to be due to stones. (It is more likely to be due to tumour.) A palpable gallbladder may be due to stones in the billiary tree or carcinoma causing obstruction.

Stones within the gallbladder cause fibrosis which results in a shrunken gallbladder which is scarred and therefore unable to dilate.

2.22   Hydatid disease   Answers: B C D E

Hydatid disease is due to *Echinococcus granulosus*. It is common in sheep-rearing areas. Man ingests the ova from earth on vegetables; the ova pass to the liver via the portal circulation and form cysts within the liver. These may be asymptomatic. The cyst wall may become calcified in which case it is visible on a plain abdominal X-ray. The clinical features include:
- obstructive jaundice
- malaise
- pruritis
- anaphylaxis.

The cyst may rupture into:
- the biliary tree producing cholangitis or jaundice
- the lung producing haemoptysis
- the peritoneum producing peritonitis
- the bowel and hence pass in the faeces.

Failed medical treatment, high risk of rupture or complications are the indications for surgery, in which the cyst is excised.

2.23   Swelling at the angle of the jaw   Answers: B D

A pharyngeal pouch is a diverticulum of the pharynx occurring at the junction between the pharynx and the oesophagus. It is due to inco-ordination of the inferior constrictor muscle during swallowing which causes a rise in the pressure within the pharynx. This results in a bulge at a weak point. The typical symptom is regurgitation of undigested food. This may cause hoarseness of the voice. The pouch presses on the oesophagus and causes dysphagia and weight loss. Chest infections may occur if food is aspirated. A swelling is rare but if present it occurs low, behind the sternocleidomastoid muscle. The diagnosis is made on barium swallow. Treatment is by surgical excision.

Enlarged lymph nodes are the commonest cause of a lump in the neck. They are due to infection or neoplasia.

A thyroglossal cyst occurs in the midline, along the thyroglossal tract. It moves on swallowing and on protrusion of the tongue.

A carotid body tumour arises in the chemoreceptor tissue at the carotid bifurcation, level with the hyoid bone. It occurs slightly lower down than a branchial cyst. It is deep to the anterior edge of the sternocleidomastoid muscle and may be pulsatile. It can be moved from side to side but not up and down. Treatment is by surgical removal.

Thyroid tissue tends to extend retrosternally, not towards the jaw.

2.24   Breast carcinoma   Answers: A D E

Breast carcinoma is the most common carcinoma in women. It commonly occurs in women aged over 40 years and the incidence increases with age. Only 1% of breast cancers occur in men. The aetiology is unknown. However, risk factors include:

- genetic factors – women who have first-degree relatives with breast/ovarian cancer are at increased risk
- environmental – there is a geographical distribution, eg there is a low incidence in Japan
- previous breast cancer – when one breast is affected the risk is increased in the other breast
- nulliparous women and those who had their first pregnancy over the age of 30 years: it is thought that oestrogens unopposed by progesterones increase susceptibility
- ionising radiation
- obesity (oestrogens are produced in peripheral fat).

Protective factors:
- early first pregnancy
- breast-feeding.

The incidence of breast carcinoma does not appear to be affected by the oral contraceptive pill.

2.25   Hydrocele   Answers: B C

A hydrocele is a serous collection of fluid within the processus vaginalis. It is idiopathic or due to trauma, infection or neoplasia. The clinical features are:
- scrotal swelling, usually without pain
- the cord is palpable above the swelling
- the testis is not palpable as it is surrounded by fluid

- it is fluctuant
- it is transilluminable
- it is irreducible.

Fertility should not be affected.

The treatment is:
- aspiration (but fluid tends to re-collect)
- surgical excision.

2.26   Scrotal swelling   Answers: C D
A hydrocele envelops the testis and the testis is usually not palpable (see Paper 2, Question 25).

A strangulated inguinal hernia may occur in the scrotum but does not transilluminate.

An encysted hydrocele of the cord in the scrotum is separate from the testis and transilluminates.

An epididymal cyst is fluid-filled and separate from the testis. Therefore the testis is palpable separately.

Epididymal tuberculosis causes swelling confined to the scrotum; there is thickening of the cord, which feels hard. It does not transilluminate.

2.27   Acute renal failure   Answers: A B C D
Post-operatively, renal failure develops in the following conditions:
- lack of renal perfusion, ie hypovolaemia due to haemorrhage or dehydration
- infection, especially Gram-negative septicaemia
- in patients who have pre-existing renal disease.

An accurate fluid chart is required to monitor fluid balance. Furosemide (frusemide) or dopamine may be used to promote diuresis. Hyperkalaemia and acidosis occur.

A renal calculus is unlikely to cause acute renal failure post-operatively (as this would have to affect both kidneys) but obstruction of the ureter may result in hydronephrosis and reduced renal function.

2.28 Extradural haemorrhage Answer: C

The classic history of an extradural haemorrhage is loss of consciousness with a 'lucid interval' before a deterioration in the Glasgow Coma Scale score. It is usually caused by damage to the middle meningeal artery. Haematoma develops between the dura and the skull, raising intracranial pressure.
The lateralising signs are an ipsilateral dilated pupil, and contralateral hemiparesis.

A skull fracture may not be present and there may not be a history of loss of consciousness.

Raised intracranial pressure causes a rise in blood pressure and a fall in heart rate. Treatment includes:
* mannitol (an osmotic diuretic)
* evacuation of haematoma via a burr hole or craniotomy.

2.29 Undescended testis Answers: C D

An undescended testis lies anywhere along the course of descent from the abdomen to the scrotum. It is usually accompanied by a congenital inguinal hernia. Most cases are recognised in infancy or childhood and should be corrected early, if possible by the age of two years. An undescended testis predisposes to malignancy. The affected testis may be small and fertility may be impaired but if the other testis is functioning normally, this prevents sterility. There is an increased risk of torsion.

2.30 Varicocele Answers: C D E

A varicocele is a collection of dilated veins of the pampiniform plexus. It is much more common on the left than on the right side. It is associated with renal tumours on the left side as this may obstruct drainage of the left testicular vein into the left renal vein.

The patient complains of a lump and/or an aching dull pain. A varicocele is likened to 'a bag of worms'. It is more noticeable when the patient is standing. It may be associated with infertility. Treatment is conservative but in troublesome cases embolisation can be performed. Alternatively, the veins can be ligated and divided.

2.31 Raynaud's phenomenon Answers: C E

Raynaud's phenomenon describes certain changes of the hands or feet occurring in response to cold. Classically the fingers first turn white due to arterial spasm and the fingers become cold. Then they turn blue due to cyanosis and finally they turn red due to reactive hyperaemia; this is painful.

Raynaud's phenomenon may be idiopathic but it is associated with:
- a cervical rib
- cervical spondylosis
- connective tissue disorders, eg rheumatoid arthritis
- oesophagitis (note that oesophagitis occurs and not oesophageal carcinoma), CREST syndrome, scleroderma and telangiectasia
- use of vibratory tools
- arterial disease, eg atherosclerosis and emboli from the subclavian artery
- drugs, eg alpha-receptor stimulants
- blood disorders, eg hyperviscosity.

2.32 Pancreatitis – complications   Answers: C E
The main complications of acute pancreatitis are:
- pseudocyst formation
- pancreatic abscess
- acute respiratory distress syndrome (ARDS)
- pleural effusions
- renal failure
- ileus – this is not due to obstruction
- shock – hypovolaemia and tachycardia
- diabetes mellitus
- metabolic effects – albumin falls, hypocalcaemia, hypomagnesaemia
- necrotising haemorrhagic pancreatitis – fat necrosis can cause embolism; also calcium is sequestered
- haemorrhage – into a pseudocyst or due to peptic ulceration.

Carcinoma of the pancreas and stones in the ampulla of Vater cause acute pancreatitis; hyperparathyroidism, hypercalcaemia and hyperlipidaemia predispose to pancreatitis.

2.33 Rodent ulcers   Answer: B
A 'rodent ulcer' is a basal cell carcinoma. It characteristically presents on the upper part of the face and ears, especially on sun-exposed areas, but can occur on the neck or anywhere else on the body. It presents as a pearly white nodule with telangiectasia. As it enlarges, it may ulcerate with a pearly rolled edge.

Basal cell carcinomas do not metastasise. They are malignant by way of their local invasion and can cause significant tissue damage by eroding into local tissue.

Treatment:
- local excision
- radiotherapy (very effective)
- cryotherapy.

2.34   Recurrent fistulae   Answers: A B C

Infection in the anorectal region can lead to abscess or fistula formation. The causes of recurrent fistulae are:
- infection (eg tuberculosis)
- Crohn's disease (anal fissures are the most common anal lesion)
- neoplasia
- ulcerative colitis
- hidradenitis suppurativa.

Diverticulitis is a common cause of fistulae in the sigmoid colon but not of the anal canal. Remember that a fistula is an abnormal tract connecting two epithelial surfaces.

2.35   Abdominal pain with hypotension   Answers: A D

Abdominal pain radiating to the back and presenting with 'shock' is a leaking abdominal aortic aneurysm until and unless proved otherwise (see Paper 1, Question 55).

There is often a history of collapse. The differential diagnosis is:
- acute pancreatitis
- mesenteric thrombosis
- myocardial infarction
- perforated peptic ulcer.

The history, examination and investigations clinch the diagnosis. It is important to make the diagnosis of a leaking abdominal aortic aneurysm promptly as it presents a surgical emergency which requires immediate transfer to theatre. Obtain:
- intravenous access with two large-bore cannulae
- blood for full blood count, urea and electrolytes, clotting screen, crossmatch for ten units of blood.

Resuscitation should maintain blood pressure but avoid overloading with fluids as this would increase the haemorrhage.

The patient requires a central line, urinary catheter and immediate surgery.

Renal colic typically presents with loin pain.

Acute appendicitis causes a localised peritonitis in the right iliac fossa. Shock occurs if the appendix perforates.

Pelvic inflammatory disease is unlikely to cause abdominal pain radiating to the back.

2.36   Tetany   Answers: A B D

Tetany is the muscle spasm that occurs in hypocalcaemia.

A metabolic alkalosis raises the pH as hydrogen ion concentration falls. This causes calcium to move into cells (hence the serum calcium level is reduced) and results in muscle twitching.

In thyroidectomy, a well-known complication is the removal of the parathyroid glands. This results in reduced parathyroid hormone and a fall in serum calcium.

A dirty wound causes tetanus, not tetany!

Over breathing causes the Pco_2 to fall, ie respiratory alkalosis. Hypocalcaemia occurs and the muscles become hyperexcitable.

Hypokalaemia is a recognised complication of paralytic ileus, not hypocalcaemia.

2.37   Ingrowing toenail   Answers: C D E

An ingrowing toenail occurs when the nail grows downwards into the soft tissue adjacent to it. It most commonly occurs on the lateral side of the big toe. It becomes infected and swollen, causing pain and discomfort. The treatment is:
- to cut the nail square and keep it clean
- antibiotics are used in the acute stage for local infection
- surgical treatment includes wedge excision of the nail and nail bed or avulsion of the nail and nail bed.

2.38   Upper gastrointestinal (GI) bleed   **Answers: D E**
Haematemesis of one litre is a medical emergency. Resuscitation is mandatory, with attention to the airway, breathing and circulation.

Intravenous access is obtained and fluid loss is replaced with blood, colloid or crystalloid. Blood should be sent for a full blood count, urea and electrolytes, clotting screen and crossmatch. Pulse rate, blood pressure, and respiratory rate are monitored. (Hypovolaemia causes low blood pressure and tachycardia.) A central venous pressure line is useful to maintain fluid balance.

Gastroscopy is performed as soon as possible (within six hours), particularly in patients over 65 years, in patients who have a postural drop in blood pressure, where there is persistent tachycardia and when haemoglobin is < 10 g/dl.

Gastroscopy is performed to identify the source of the blood loss and facilitates treatment such as injection sclerotherapy. Surgery is indicated in persistent bleeding.

2.39   Pilonidal sinus   **Answers: A D E**
A pilonidal sinus is a sinus containing hairs. It commonly occurs in hair-bearing areas and may become infected to produce a pilonidal abscess. The commonest site is the natal cleft but it is also seen in the fingers of hairdressers where hairs become implanted under the skin. A pilonidal sinus tends to persist, with chronic discharge via one or more sinuses to the skin. Treatment is by excision of the sinus with surrounding tissue.

2.40   Malignant melanoma   **Answers: A B C**
Malignant melanoma is a malignant tumour of melanocytes. It commonly occurs on the soles of the feet and on the head and neck. It can occur in the nail bed, eye or mouth. Malignant melanoma is associated with exposure to ultraviolet light. The highest incidence is seen in Queensland, Australia. The incidence is lower in black populations.

Most tumours are pigmented but some have no pigment, ie they are amelanotic. Changes in the appearance of a mole should arouse suspicion. Malignant melanomas itch, bleed and ulcerate.

Some undergo spontaneous regression but this is not associated with hypophysectomy.

The treatment of choice is surgery, with wide local excision of the lesion. Radiotherapy and chemotherapy are used for palliation in cases that have spread.

2.41   Buerger's disease   Answers: A B C E

Buerger's disease affects young men who smoke. It affects all limbs. The arteries become obliterated, resulting in ischaemia of the affected areas. The veins and nerves are also affected. Patients present with peripheral ischaemic disease resulting in ulcers and digital gangrene. The treatment is to **stop smoking**. Otherwise, progressive ischaemia occurs with gangrene, and amputation becomes necessary.

2.42   Carotid artery stenosis   Answers: A B D

Carotid artery occlusion usually occurs at the carotid bifurcation. It often goes unnoticed because the brain receives a contralateral blood supply via the circle of Willis.

Patients present with transient ischaemic attacks causing weakness in the contralateral limbs or amaurosis fugax which is a transient loss of vision in the ipsilateral eye. These resolve within a few hours. The cause is emboli from the carotid circulation impacting in smaller intracerebral vessels.

Vomiting is not a sign of carotid disease. It would indicate disease of the posterior circulation.

Patients with symptoms and stenosis greater than 70% should be treated with endarterectomy.

2.43   Anal fissure   Answers: A B D

The treatment of anal fissures may be:
*   **conservative** – with laxatives and local anaesthetic agents, some fissures heal spontaneously
*   **surgical** – this is either by 'anal dilatation' or 'lateral sphincterotomy'.

Surgery is indicated in cases of persistent fissures which become chronic. At surgery, examination under anaesthesia is performed to exclude other pathology. In Crohn's disease, sphincterotomy is not advised as there is a risk of sepsis.

2.44   Carpal tunnel syndrome   **Answers: C D E**
Carpal tunnel syndrome is caused by compression of the median nerve in
the carpal tunnel, deep to the flexor retinaculum.

The median nerve supplies the 'LOAF' muscles:
  Lumbricals I & II
  Oponens pollicis
  Abductor pollicis brevis
  Flexor pollicis

These are the muscles of the thenar eminence.

Carpal tunnel syndrome causes wasting of the thenar eminence (the ulnar
nerve supplies the muscles of the hypothenar eminence) and weakness of
these muscles. Sensory loss occurs in the lateral three and a half fingers.
Patients complain of paraesthesia especially in this distribution. There is
pain in the forearm which is often worse at night.

On continuous tapping over the flexor retinaculum the pain may be
reproduced – this is Tinel's sign. Pain may also be reproduced by flexion
of the wrist for 1–2 minutes – this is Phalen's sign.

Application of a tourniquet inflated to greater than arterial pressure may
also reproduce the symptoms.

Surgical treatment involves division of the flexor retinaculum.

2.45   Compound fracture of a bone   **Answers: B C**
A compound fracture is also known as an 'open fracture'. It is a fracture of
a bone with breach of the overlying tissue, allowing access to the exterior.
This poses a major risk of infection.

The first-line treatment is:
• to cover the wound with an iodine-soaked dressing
• antibiotic prophylaxis with penicillin and flucloxacillin
• tetanus immunisation
• debridement
• skeletal stabilisation.

Operative fixation may be carried out at this stage.

2.46   H$_2$ antagonists   **Answers: A C D**

Ranitidine is an H$_2$ antagonist. It acts by blocking the histamine receptors in the stomach, thereby reducing gastric acid secretion. Cimetidine is another example. Both may be given orally or intravenously. They may be used immediately in upper gastrointestinal bleeding and are also useful in the prevention of stress ulcers of which there is risk in major operations.

2.47   Peptic ulcers   **Answers: B C E**

Peptic ulcers are ulcers of the stomach and duodenum.

The emergency complications are haemorrhage, perforation and pyloric stenosis.

Haemorrhage is due to erosion of the mucosa and blood vessel walls.

Perforation occurs when erosion of the bowel goes through the full thickness of the bowel wall.

Chronic ulceration may result in stricture formation due to fibrosis. This may occur in the body of the stomach, pylorus or duodenum.

Peptic ulcers are associated with:
* cigarette smoking
* stress
* genetic factors (eg where there is a family history)
* hyperparathyroidism – calcium levels are raised which stimulates gastric acid secretion.

Hyperparathyroidism presents with:
* abdominal pain
* bone disease:
  – subperiosteal erosions visible on X-ray
  – small lytic lesions of the skull (pepperpot skull)
  – cystic lesions of bone
* renal calculi (ie 'stones, bones and abdominal groans!')
* drugs, eg aspirin, steroids and non-steroidal anti-inflammatory drugs (NSAIDs)
* post-renal transplant
* Meckel's diverticulum – may contain ectopic gastric mucosa which secretes gastrin
* Zollinger–Ellison syndrome.

2.48 Ulcerative colitis versus Crohn's disease   Answers: A D

Feature	Ulcerative colitis	Crohn's disease
Rectal bleeding	+ + +	+
Diarrhoea	+ + +	+
Steatorrhoea and malabsorption	–	+ + +
Rectal involvement	+ + +	+
Abdominal mass	+ / –	+ +
Perianal lesions	+ / –	+ + +
Fistulae	+ / –	+ + +
Toxic megacolon	+ +	+ / –
Malignant change	+ +	+ / –

2.49 Dupuytren's contracture   Answers: A B

Dupuytren's contracture (or cord) is a contracture of the palmar fascia. The cause is idiopathic but there is a familial component (autosomal dominant inheritance).

A flexor deformity of the finger develops which may be debilitating. It may occur bilaterally. Cord excision is indicated if it affects daily life.

2.50 Femoral shaft fracture   Answers: A B D

The femur is a large bone and its fracture involves a considerable amount of trauma. Blood loss into the surrounding soft tissue is significant and may result in shock. Intravenous fluid replacement is required.

In closed fractures, fat embolism (from bone marrow) is a common complication.

Tetanus immunisation is mandatory in open fractures.

Internal fixation of the femur is by intramedullary nailing.

Healing of the femur takes at least three months.

2.51   Post-operative oliguria   Answers: C D

Urinary retention is a common post-operative complication occurring within 24 hours, especially in men. Examination of the abdomen is appropriate to look for an enlarged bladder. A urinary catheter may then be inserted and is diagnostic as well as therapeutic. Poor urine output may also be due to hypovolaemia. This is assessed with a fluid challenge of 200 ml, given intravenously, which should raise urine output. If there is no response, 40 mg of furosemide (frusemide), a loop diuretic, can be given. However, furosemide can be nephrotoxic and therefore care must be taken where renal failure is suspected. Persistent hypovolaemia causes acute renal failure. With rehydration, dopamine may be required to stimulate renal function. Mannitol is an osmotic diuretic and would not be appropriate. Haemodialysis can be used in the late stages.

2.52   Cellulitis   Answer: C

Cellulitis is inflammation of subcutaneous tissue which spreads locally. It is usually caused by *Streptococcus pyogenes*. The area of skin is typically red, hot and tender. Spreading cellulitis requires treatment with antibiotics, (such as intravenous penicillin). Localised infection may lead to a collection of pus in the form of an abscess which requires incision and drainage.

2.53   Meckel's diverticulum   Answers: B D E

Meckel's diverticulum is present in 2% of the population. It is the embryological remnant of the vitello-intestinal duct, and is situated on the ileum approximately two feet from the ileocaecal junction. It is not the appendix.

Aide-mémoire: RULE OF TWOs – 2%, 2 feet, and 2 inches long

It may contain gastrin-secreting mucosa which stimulates acid secretion by the stomach and results in peptic ulceration.

If a Meckel's diverticulum becomes obstructed it gives rise to inflammation and presents with the features of acute appendicitis.

A Meckel's diverticulum may become inverted and cause intussusception which presents as small bowel obstruction.

2.54   Salivary duct calculi   **Answers: B C D**

The aetiology of salivary duct calculi is unknown. They are more common in the submandibular duct than in the parotid duct. The acute inflammation of the salivary glands occurring in mumps is more common in the parotid gland.)

The calculi cause obstruction of the duct and stasis of saliva, which increases the risk of infection. Clinically, the features are:
* painful swelling of the gland which is usually unilateral
* pain on eating meals as saliva production increases
* a foul taste in the mouth
* sudden relief of symptoms.

The standard investigations are plain X-rays and sialography. Submandibular duct calculi tend to be quite large and are therefore calcified. This shows up on X-ray. Parotid duct calculi, however, tend to be small and are often radiolucent.

An ultrasound scan is useful to diagnose an abscess.

2.55   Carcinoma of the stomach   **Answers: B C D E**

Carcinoma of the stomach is common. It occurs in men more often than in women, in a ratio of 2:1. It is most common in the antrum. It may occur as a result of malignant transformation of a polyp or as a primary lesion. The symptoms include epigastric pain, loss of appetite, loss of weight, dysphagia, regurgitation and vomiting. The patient appears cachectic. An epigastric mass may be palpable, with tenderness and obstruction. Fluid in the stomach causes a succussion splash. There may be iron deficiency and/or pernicious anaemia. Metastases occur:
* by local invasion
* via lymphatics:
  - to the liver, causing ascites, hepatomegaly and jaundice
  - to the lungs, causing pleural effusions
  - to the brain
  - to lymph nodes (an enlarged lymph node in the left supraclavicular fossa is called Virchow's node or Troisier's sign)
* via the bloodstream
* by transcoelomic spread.

Metastases to the ovaries cause 'Krukenberg tumours'.

Surgical treatment is gastrectomy – total or partial, but the recurrence rate in the remnant is significant.

Prognosis depends on the extent of spread. In general, patients tend to present late and therefore prognosis is poor – a five-year survival rate of 10–25%.

2.56   Ureteric calculi   **Answers: A D**
The symptoms of ureteric calculi include loin pain which is colicky or constant, radiating into the groin and scrotum. The patient may roll about in pain with little relief. Microscopic or macroscopic haematuria occurs.

Approximately 70% of stones contain calcium oxalate; 15% are mixed phosphate stones; and 8% are uric acid.

'Triple phosphate' stones are composed of calcium, magnesium and ammonium phosphate. This forms the typical 'staghorn calculus'. It is caused by the urease-producing organism, *Proteus*.

Stone formation is increased in:
• hyperparathyroidism (increased calcium)
• gout
• cystinuria.

Urinary stasis predisposes to the precipitation of crystals and stone formation.

Infection producing alkaline urine causes the precipitation of calcium.

Schistosomiasis predisposes to bladder calculi.

Treatment includes:
• analgesia, eg diclofenac, for symptomatic relief
• lithotripsy
• ureteroscopic removal
• surgery.

Ureteric calculi do not predispose to transitional cell carcinoma of the ureter.

Bladder calculi cause irritation and an increased incidence of bladder tumours of the squamous cell type.

2.57   Metabolic response to trauma   Answers: B C E

Remember that trauma refers to all types of injury, whether accidental or surgical. The physiological response occurs in two phases:

- the **ebb phase** – this occurs in the first 24 hours. During this time there is:
  - increased sympathetic activity
  - increased acute phase proteins
  - energy reserves are mobilised (glucose and triglyceride levels increase)
  - insulin secretion decreases
  - adrenocorticotrophin hormone (ACTH) increases – this causes a rise in cortisol levels and thus sodium and water retention with potassium loss
  - release of antidiuretic hormone (ADH) to maintain blood pressure by fluid retention

- the **flow phase** – this occurs days to weeks later:
  - metabolic rate is increased
  - nitrogen excretion is increased due to protein catabolism – protein loss occurs from skeletal muscle breakdown, resulting in loss of lean body mass
  - energy is consumed
  - insulin resistance occurs.

2.58   Rectal bleeding – bright red   Answers: B E

The passage of bright red blood with the stool is usually due to local pathology.

Haemorrhoids are a common cause. However, a thrombosed pile consists of solid clot and altered blood which is dark red. Therefore, fresh red bleeding does not occur.

Anal fissure – constipation causes trauma to the fissure which opens up and causes bleeding.

Neoplasia, for example adenoma or carcinoma of the rectum: these are situated close to the anal margin and can cause fresh red bleeding. More proximal colonic carcinoma would cause blood to be mixed in with the stool.

Trauma – local injury.

Note that the question specifies 'bright red blood' but there are numerous other causes of rectal bleeding (see also Paper 3, Question 55).

An ischiorectal abscess occurs in the ischiorectal fossa, the main symptom being pain.

2.59   Staging of breast carcinoma   **Answers: A B**
Staging of breast tumours is used to assess spread, predict prognosis and facilitate treatment.

Diagnosis is made by:
- ultrasound scan
- mammography
- fine-needle aspiration or biopsy
- lumpectomy.

Staging is done using the TNM classification:
- T = tumour size and extent (T_0–T_4; Tis representing 'carcinoma in situ')
- N = spread to lymph nodes (N_0–N_3)
- M = metastases (M_0 or M_1, indicating the presence or absence of metastases).

Stage	Features	Five-year survival
I	Tumour ≤ 2 cm	85%
II	Tumour ≤ 5 cm Nodes not fixed	65%
III	Tumour ≤ 5 cm Supraclavicular nodes fixed	40%
IV	Distant metastases	10%

The Manchester system of staging is as follows:
Treatment: in localized disease, ie for stages I and II, surgery is indicated. This includes wide local excision, axillary clearance and adjuvant radiotherapy or chemotherapy.

If metastases are present, ie stages III and IV, treatment is palliative, with radiotherapy and drugs, for example tamoxifen, corticosteroids and chemotherapy.

2.60   Hypocalcaemia   **Answers: C E**

Calcium is present largely in bones; a small amount is present in blood, both as ions and bound to albumin. If acidity [H^+] increases, free calcium ions increase. Calcium levels must be corrected with respect to albumin as follows:

Corrected calcium = measured calcium + (40 – albumin) x 0.02

Calcium levels depend on intake and loss.

The causes of hypocalcaemia are:
- hypoparathyroidism
- chronic renal failure
- vitamin D deficiency
- septicaemia
- acute pancreatitis (gallstones can cause this but do not cause hypocalcaemia directly).

In thyroidectomy, a complication is removal of the parathyroid glands which results in hypocalcaemia.

In low calcium states, replacement is with intravenous calcium gluconate.

In multiple myeloma and other malignancy, calcium levels tend to be raised. Parathyroid adenoma causes hypercalcaemia due to excess parathyroid hormone secretion.

MULTIPLE CHOICE QUESTION PAPER 3

60 questions: time allowed 2½ hours.
Mark your answers with a tick (True) or a cross (False) in the box provided.
Leave the box blank for 'Don't know'. Do not look at the answers until you
have completed the whole question paper.

3.1 Colles' fracture

- ❏ A requires manipulation of the humerus with immobilisation for six weeks
- ❏ B may lead to delayed rupture of extensor pollicis longus
- ❏ C can be manipulated under local anaesthesia
- ❏ D occurs following a fall onto the outstretched hand
- ❏ E usually unites in six weeks

3.2 Epistaxis

- ❏ A is bleeding from the epiglottis
- ❏ B usually occurs from Little's area
- ❏ C can cause a drop in blood pressure
- ❏ D can be treated with nasal packing
- ❏ E may require internal carotid artery ligation

3.3 Laparoscopic cholecystectomy

- ❏ A is routinely performed for elective cholecystectomy
- ❏ B has the advantage of small incisions, compared to open cholecystectomy
- ❏ C has no complications
- ❏ D is contraindicated in the elderly
- ❏ E is used for appendicitis

3.4 Hypercalcaemia causes

- ❏ A renal stones
- ❏ B polyuria
- ❏ C constipation
- ❏ D gallstones
- ❏ E tetanus

3.5 Acute extradural haemorrhage

- [ ] A causes a rise in pulse rate and a fall in blood pressure
- [ ] B causes a fall in pulse rate and a rise in blood pressure
- [ ] C results in hemiparesis
- [ ] D is associated with a dilated pupil on the side of the injury
- [ ] E can be distinguished from subdural haemorrhage by CT scan

3.6 Carcinoma of the caecum

- [ ] A presents early with bloody diarrhoea
- [ ] B is treated by right hemicolectomy
- [ ] C is associated with microcytic anaemia
- [ ] D is associated with Crohn's disease
- [ ] E is diagnosed with sigmoidoscopy

3.7 A supracondylar fracture of the humerus may lead to

- [ ] A injury to the brachial artery
- [ ] B injury to the ulnar nerve
- [ ] C avascular necrosis of the radius
- [ ] D injury of the axillary artery
- [ ] E infarction of forearm muscles

3.8 Gallstone ileus

- [ ] A causes large bowel obstruction
- [ ] B causes small bowel obstruction
- [ ] C is due to lack of contraction of the gallbladder
- [ ] D may result in an abdominal X-ray showing gas in the biliary tree
- [ ] E is treated by cholecystostomy

3.9 Blood transfusion

- [ ] A reaction may manifest as pruritis
- [ ] B should be stopped if pyrexia develops
- [ ] C blood is screened for hepatitis B antibody
- [ ] D reactions are most often due to blood mismatch
- [ ] E reaction may lead to jaundice

3.10 A swelling with an expansile pulsation above the left clavicle may be

- ❏ A a Pancoast tumour
- ❏ B an aneurysm of the subclavian artery
- ❏ C a dilated subclavian vein
- ❏ D a Virchow's node
- ❏ E a branchial cyst

3.11 Features consistent with a diagnosis of acute ulcerative colitis include

- ❏ A a normal barium enema
- ❏ B tachycardia > 100/minute
- ❏ C weight gain
- ❏ D serum albumin < 30 g/l
- ❏ E dilatation of the colon on plain abdominal X-ray

3.12 Which of the following occur in anterior perforation of peptic ulcers

- ❏ A board-like rigidity
- ❏ B an increased area of liver dullness to percussion
- ❏ C a state of collapse dominating the picture shortly after onset
- ❏ D gas under the diaphragm on an erect chest X-ray
- ❏ E peritonitis

3.13 Colonic polyps

- ❏ A may be benign
- ❏ B may be malignant
- ❏ C should be left untreated if asymptomatic
- ❏ D of the tubular type in the colon are less likely to undergo malignant change than the villous type
- ❏ E may occur in Peutz–Jeghers syndrome

3.14   Crohn's disease

❑   A   is associated with finger clubbing
❑   B   may cause protein malabsorption
❑   C   is characteristically associated with dilatation of the terminal ileum
❑   D   hardly ever affects the colon
❑   E   may undergo spontaneous symptomatic remission

3.15   Which of the following symptoms and signs are suggestive of paralytic ileus

❑   A   abdominal distension
❑   B   hyperactive bowel sounds
❑   C   vomiting
❑   D   colicky abdominal pain
❑   E   gas and fluid levels in dilated loops of small bowel on X-ray

3.16   Dysphagia

❑   A   means difficulty in swallowing
❑   B   means difficulty in speaking
❑   C   may occur in a patient who has had a stroke
❑   D   is associated with carcinoma of the oesophagus
❑   E   occurs in pyloric stenosis

3.17   Diverticular disease of the colon

❑   A   may present with pneumaturia
❑   B   always occurs in the jejunum
❑   C   is common in Western societies
❑   D   may present with massive bleeding
❑   E   is a causative factor in the development of carcinoma of the colon

3.18   A femoral hernia

❑   A   should be treated with a truss
❑   B   has the femoral vein lateral to it
❑   C   may contain omentum
❑   D   appears above and medial to the inguinal ligament
❑   E   can strangulate the bowel without obstructing it

3.19   **In the radiological differentiation between cancer of the colon and diverticulitis, which of the following features would favour a diagnosis of diverticulitis**

- ❏   A   a long segment of affected bowel
- ❏   B   an abrupt transition from abnormal to normal bowel
- ❏   C   evidence of spasm of the colon
- ❏   D   diverticula
- ❏   E   apple-core appearance

3.20   **Sequelae of acute cholecystitis include**

- ❏   A   a perforation of the gallbladder
- ❏   B   cholecystoduodenal fistula
- ❏   C   ascending cholecystitis
- ❏   D   an enlarged palpable gallbladder
- ❏   E   septicaemia

3.21   **Hepatitis B**

- ❏   A   is transmitted by the faeco-oral route
- ❏   B   vaccine should be given to 'at risk' healthcare workers
- ❏   C   predisposes to hepatocellular carcinoma
- ❏   D   may cause liver cirrhosis
- ❏   E   is an RNA virus

3.22   **Ascending cholangitis is associated with**

- ❏   A   large bowel obstruction
- ❏   B   gallstones
- ❏   C   fever
- ❏   D   stricture of the common bile duct
- ❏   E   cholangiocarcinoma

3.23   **Carcinoma of the oesophagus**

- ❏   A   is diagnosed at colonoscopy
- ❏   B   presents with dysuria
- ❏   C   spreads to the liver
- ❏   D   can be treated with radiotherapy
- ❏   E   can be treated with surgery

3.24   A breast lump that is fixed to skin but not to deep tissues may be

❑   A   a fibroadenoma
❑   B   a cyst
❑   C   an intraduct papilloma
❑   D   an abscess
❑   E   fat necrosis

3.25   Clinical findings of a ruptured spleen may include

❑   A   haemorrhagic shock
❑   B   haematemesis
❑   C   reduced bowel sounds
❑   D   abdominal distension
❑   E   shifting dullness within the abdomen

3.26   Predisposing factors in the formation of renal calculi are

❑   A   Dupuytren's contracture
❑   B   a tropical climate
❑   C   thyrotoxicosis
❑   D   parathyroid tumour
❑   E   malnutrition

3.27   In a case of abdominal trauma followed by haematuria

❑   A   the kidney should be explored immediately
❑   B   an intravenous urogram is of no value
❑   C   a CT scan of the abdomen should be obtained
❑   D   nephrectomy may be required
❑   E   the patient must be followed up

3.28   Regarding ulcerative colitis

❑   A   malignancy is a feature
❑   B   transmural involvement occurs
❑   C   the rectum is always involved
❑   D   it is familial
❑   E   crypt abscesses are seen

3.29   A direct inguinal hernia

- ❏   A   is usually congenital
- ❏   B   may contain bowel, omentum or bladder
- ❏   C   may occur with an indirect hernia
- ❏   D   protrudes through the posterior wall of the inguinal canal, lateral to the inferior epigastric vessels
- ❏   E   has a high risk of strangulation

3.30   Recognised complications of venous insufficiency of the lower limb include

- ❏   A   chronic ulceration
- ❏   B   superficial phlebitis
- ❏   C   stiffness of the ankle joint
- ❏   D   deep vein thrombosis
- ❏   E   localized eczema

3.31   Digital gangrene may be caused by

- ❏   A   frostbite
- ❏   B   alcoholism
- ❏   C   ergot derivatives
- ❏   D   polyneuritis
- ❏   E   cervical rib

3.32   In pancreatitis

- ❏   A   antibiotics are mandatory
- ❏   B   the clinical picture is a reliable indicator of prognosis
- ❏   C   treatment is conservative
- ❏   D   laparotomy may be indicated
- ❏   E   a rise in serum amylase is diagnostic

3.33   A carbuncle

- ❏   A   is associated with glycosuria
- ❏   B   is commonly found on the palm of the hand
- ❏   C   is commonly found on the neck
- ❏   D   forms an area of necrosis with multiple sinuses
- ❏   E   is best treated with systemic antibiotics

3.34   An anal fissure

❏   A   is associated with a sentinel pile
❏   B   most commonly lies anteriorly
❏   C   is an ulcer of the rectal mucosa
❏   D   is a cause of bleeding in infancy
❏   E.   is a recognised complication of Crohn's disease

3.35   The effect of an arterial embolus depends on

❏   A   collateral circulation of the area where the embolus lodges
❏   B   site of origin
❏   C   size of the embolus
❏   D   composition of the embolus
❏   E   time of onset of thrombolysis

3.36   Coronary artery grafting for ischaemic heart disease

❏   A   always requires cardiopulmonary bypass
❏   B   is usually performed using intercostal arteries as grafts
❏   C   is unlikely to be successful if more than two major coronary
          arteries are narrowed
❏   D   requires preceding coronary angiography
❏   E   has not been shown to prolong life

**3.37   The following are proved methods of prophylaxis in reducing
          the incidence of deep vein thrombosis:**

❏   A   pneumatic calf compression during operations
❏   B   subcutaneous low molecular weight heparin daily
❏   C   elasticated compression stockings
❏   D   aspirin 300 mg four times a day
❏   E   immobilisation

3.38   Surgical emphysema may be caused by

❏   A   spontaneous pneumothorax
❏   B   perforation of the oesophagus
❏   C   hyperventilation
❏   D   traumatic pneumothorax
❏   E   smoking

3.39   Anal pain occurs in

- ❏ A   carcinoma of the anal canal
- ❏ B   first-degree haemorrhoids
- ❏ C   anal fissure
- ❏ D   anal warts
- ❏ E   perianal haematoma

3.40   The following apply to malignant melanoma

- ❏ A   they usually arise from a pre-existing mole
- ❏ B   the prognosis depends on the depth of invasion
- ❏ C   the prognosis is worse in the superficial spreading form than in the nodular form
- ❏ D   the prognosis is worse in amelanotic lesions
- ❏ E   they metastasise to regional lymph nodes

3.41   The following are features of peripheral arterial disease

- ❏ A   intermittent claudication
- ❏ B   transient ischaemic attacks
- ❏ C   diabetes mellitus
- ❏ D   rest pain
- ❏ E   critical ischaemia

3.42   Infection with tuberculosis produces

- ❏ A   a hot red abscess
- ❏ B   granuloma formation
- ❏ C   collapse of vertebral bodies
- ❏ D   epididymitis
- ❏ E   frequency of micturition

3.43   Carcinoma of the tongue

- ❏ A   is associated with constipation
- ❏ B   usually occurs on the posterior third
- ❏ C   is associated with the presence of leukoplakia
- ❏ D   is usually an adenocarcinoma
- ❏ E   may be treated by radiotherapy

3.44   A prolapsed lumbar intervertebral disc

❏ A   presents with arm pain
❏ B   may cause urinary retention
❏ C   at the level of L3/4 may result in an absent knee jerk
❏ D   may present with buttock pain
❏ E   may be treated conservatively

3.45   Metastases in bone are a common feature of carcinoma of the

❏ A   kidney
❏ B   rectum
❏ C   lungs
❏ D   stomach
❏ E   thyroid

3.46   Heparin

❏ A   is given intravenously in the prophylaxis of deep vein thrombosis
❏ B   may cause osteomalacia
❏ C   is reversible with protamine
❏ D   has a half-life of 12 hours
❏ E   action is monitored by the international normalized ratio

3.47   Regarding an intertrochanteric fracture of the femur

❏ A   it is common in young men
❏ B   the leg is shortened and externally rotated
❏ C   it is treated with internal fixation
❏ D   there is a high risk of avascular necrosis of the head of the femur
❏ E   it should be treated with total hip replacement

3.48   Concerning antibiotics

❏ A   a cephalosporin is used prophylactically in cholecystectomy
❏ B   a complete course should be given for prophylaxis in surgery
❏ C   they are the treatment of choice for an abscess
❏ D   prophylaxis is advised for surgery in patients with prosthetic heart valves
❏ E   prophylaxis is recommended in colorectal surgery

3.49 **Which of the following are complications of urinary catheterisation**

❑ A   renal stones
❑ B   chronic pyelonephritis
❑ C   septicaemia
❑ D   prostatitis
❑ E   urethral bleeding

3.50 **Hyperhidrosis**

❑ A   is dryness of the skin
❑ B   is associated with an increase in the number of eccrine glands
❑ C   does not occur in the palms
❑ D   can be eliminated by a sympathectomy
❑ E   classically affects young women

3.51 **Before starting an urgent operation for large bowel obstruction which of the following investigations should be carried out**

❑ A   full blood count
❑ B   chest X-ray
❑ C   barium enema
❑ D   sigmoidoscopy
❑ E   electrolyte concentrations in serum

3.52 **Pseudomembranous colitis**

❑ A   is caused by *Clostridium perfringens*
❑ B   may occur after only one dose of an antibiotic
❑ C   may occur weeks after antibiotic treatment
❑ D   may occur after treatment with cephalosporins
❑ E   is treated with intravenous metronidazole

3.53 **In the first 12 hours following a major abdominal operation, particular attention should be paid to**

❑ A   urinary output
❑ B   pupil size
❑ C   wound drainage
❑ D   respiration
❑ E   core temperature

3.54 Total parenteral nutrition

- ❏ A is beneficial for most malnourished patients pre-operatively
- ❏ B is beneficial for malnourished patients post-operatively
- ❏ C is usually given via a peripheral intravenous line
- ❏ D carries a risk of sepsis
- ❏ E can be given via a nasogastric tube

3.55 Blood may be found on the glove following rectal examination in

- ❏ A diverticulitis
- ❏ B Meckel's diverticulum
- ❏ C carcinoma of the oesophagus
- ❏ D intussusception
- ❏ E chronic prostatitis

3.56 Thyroid carcinoma

- ❏ A of the papillary type usually affects young adults
- ❏ B presents as a lump in the neck that moves on swallowing
- ❏ C of the anaplastic type carries the best prognosis
- ❏ D of the medullary type is a tumour of parafollicular cells
- ❏ E typically causes thyroid dysfunction

3.57 Regarding kidney transplant

- ❏ A it is only offered to patients under 50 years of age
- ❏ B the transplant is placed extraperitoneally
- ❏ C urine output is monitored to detect rejection
- ❏ D immunosuppression is required
- ❏ E a urinary tract infection is a contraindication

3.58 The causes of stricture of the bowel include

- ❏ A gluten enteropathy
- ❏ B slow-release potassium tablets
- ❏ C mesenteric ischaemia
- ❏ D Crohn's disease
- ❏ E Peutz–Jeghers syndrome

3.59 **The level of amylase in serum is typically raised in patients with**

❏ A acute pancreatitis
❏ B acute appendicitis
❏ C renal failure
❏ D perforated peptic ulcer
❏ E acute cholecystitis

3.60 **Volvulus**

❏ A causes venous infarction of the bowel
❏ B causes peritonitis
❏ C can be cured by performing a barium enema
❏ D occurs only in the sigmoid colon
❏ E commonly occurs in children and young adults

———————————— **END** ————————————

Go over your answers until your time is up.
Correct answers and teaching notes are overleaf.

MULTIPLE CHOICE QUESTION PAPER 3 – ANSWERS

The correct answer options for each question are given below.

3.1	B C D E		3.31	A C E
3.2	B C D		3.32	C D
3.3	A B		3.33	A C D E
3.4	A B C		3.34	A D E
3.5	C D E		3.35	A C D E
3.6	B C		3.36	D
3.7	A E		3.37	A B C
3.8	B D		3.38	B D
3.9	A E		3.39	A C E
3.10	B		3.40	B D E
3.11	B D E		3.41	A B D E
3.12	A C D E		3.42	B C D E
3.13	A B D		3.43	C E
3.14	A B E		3.44	B C D E
3.15	A C E		3.45	A C E
3.16	A C D		3.46	C
3.17	A C D		3.47	B C
3.18	B C E		3.48	A D E
3.19	A C D		3.49	C D E
3.20	A B D E		3.50	D E
3.21	B C D		3.51	A B E
3.22	B C D E		3.52	B C D
3.23	C D E		3.53	A C D E
3.24	D E		3.54	B D
3.25	A C D E		3.55	A B D
3.26	B D E		3.56	A B D
3.27	C D E		3.57	B C D E
3.28	A C E		3.58	B C D
3.29	B C		3.59	A C D E
3.30	A B C E		3.60	A B C

MCQ PAPER 3 – ANSWERS AND TEACHING NOTES

3.1   Colles' fracture   **Answers: B C D E**

Colles' fracture is a transverse fracture of the distal radius (+/– ulna) resulting in a 'dinner fork' deformity of the wrist. Displacement of the distal fragment requires treatment with manipulation of the wrist under anaesthesia, to align the radius (and ulna if involved).

Extensor pollicis longus may undergo delayed rupture, possibly due to damage over the edge of the fractured radius.

Local anaesthesia can be used for a haematoma block or regional block, facilitating manipulation. A fall onto the outstretched hand is the classic history for Colles' fracture, and it commonly occurs in elderly women who have osteoporosis.

A plaster is applied to immobilise the distal radius and ulna while the fracture unites in about six weeks.

3.2   Epistaxis   **Answers: B C D**

Epistaxis is bleeding from the nose. The most common site of bleeding is from the Little's area in the anterior part of the nasal septum. The causes include nose blowing/picking, hypertension, trauma, blood disorders, neoplasia. Continuous bleeding can cause a drop in blood pressure with tachycardia. Appropriate resuscitation is required and the bleeding must be controlled.

Treatment of epistaxis includes:
* nasal packing
* blood pressure control. Hypertension can cause small blood vessels to rupture and therefore requires control
* cauterisation
* balloon catheter tamponade
* vascular ligation in life-threatening cases (external carotid artery).

3.3   Laparoscopic cholecystectomy   **Answers: A B**

Acute cholecystitis is treated with antibiotics and analgesia. Laparoscopic cholecystectomy can be performed in the acute stage or electively, usually six weeks after the acute episode has settled.

The main advantage is the small wound, resulting in an early return to daily activity. The hospital stay is shorter.

Every operation has potential complications. These should be considered as general and specific. The complications related to laparoscopic cholecystectomy are:

- **operative**
  - bowel injuries
  - vascular damage/bleeding
  - tension pneumothorax
  - biliary tract injury
  - gallstone spillage
- **post-operative**
  - bleeding
  - biliary leak
  - retained stones
  - pain
- **late**
  - incisional hernia.

The absolute contraindication is bleeding diathesis. The relative contra-indications are:

- obesity
- pregnancy
- severe cardiac morbidity
- previous abdominal surgery

Age is not a contraindication. In fact laparoscopic surgery can be very useful in the elderly.

Laparoscopic cholecystectomy is obviously not used for appendicitis. Appendicectomy is increasingly being performed laparoscopically.

3.4   Hypercalcaemia   Answers: A B C
Hypercalcaemia produces the following:
- polyuria
- polydipsia
- fatigue
- constipation
- bone pain
- urinary tract stones
- abdominal pain
- pancreatitis.

Confusion and coma may also occur.

Excess calcium is excreted by the kidneys and therefore leads to the formation of renal stones. In hyperparathyroidism parathyroid hormone causes reduced calcium excretion and increased phosphate excretion. The phosphate precipitates as calcium salts and paradoxically forms renal stones.

Gallstones are formed mainly of cholesterol and/or bile, with calcium salts being a feature of both.

Constipation is a sign of both hypocalcaemia and hypercalcaemia. A fall in plasma calcium increases neuromuscular excitability, causing cramps and tetany. Paraesthesiae occur, especially of the face. Clinically, tapping over the parotid gland causes twitching – Chvostek's sign, and inflating a sphygmomanometer cuff on the arm causes carpal spasm – Trousseau's sign.

Hypocalcaemia occurs in pancreatitis and post-operatively in thyroidectomy patients if the parathyroid glands are affected.

3.5   Acute extradural haemorrhage   Answers: C D E
Extradural haemorrhage arises from injury to the middle meningeal artery, causing an extradural collection of blood.

It is usually due to a head injury, typically producing a 'lucid interval' and then deterioration in conscious level.

Intracranial pressure rises as the bleed is contained within the skull. The clinical features are headache, vomiting, papilloedema, altered conscious

level, fits and coma.
The localising signs include:
- dilated pupil on the side of the injury
- hemiparesis
- hemiplegia.

Blood pressure falls and the heart rate increases in hypovolaemia. Blood pressure rises and the heart rate falls in raised intracranial pressure.

A CT scan is diagnostic and very useful in differentiating between subdural and extradural haemorrhage.

Treatment is by urgent evaluation of the haematoma via a burr hole, or craniotomy and control of the bleeding point.

3.6   Carcinoma of the caecum   Answers: B C

Colorectal carcinoma is common, more than 70% occurring in the distal half of the colon. The sigmoid colon is the most common site. Only about 10% occur in the caecum.

Predisposing conditions are ulcerative colitis, familial adenomatous polyposis (FAP) and hereditary non-polyposis colon cancer (HNPCC).

Right-sided colonic tumours present with microcytic anaemia (iron deficiency) due to occult bleeding, a mass in the right iliac fossa and diarrhoea. They rarely cause obstruction. Systemic effects are weight loss, malaise and jaundice/hepatomegaly if liver metastases are present. The treatment for a right-sided tumour is a right hemicolectomy. The treatment for a left-sided tumour is a left hemicolectomy or sigmoid colectomy.

Rectal tumours are treated by anterior resection or abdominal-perineal resection of the rectum. Investigations include the following:
- barium enema, which may show an obvious lesion
- colonoscopy – required to visualise caecal tumours and, in addition, has the advantage of obtaining a biopsy. Synchronous tumours can be excluded. Sigmoidoscopy is not sufficient to diagnose caecal lesions. The sigmoidoscope only reaches the splenic flexure
- CT scan – will demonstrate the tumour, determine liver metastases and allow staging of the disease.

3.7   A supracondylar fracture of the humerus   Answers: A E

Supracondylar fractures are most commonly seen in children. The humerus breaks just above the condyles and the broken edge damages the soft tissues, particularly the brachial artery and median nerve. The brachial artery may go into severe spasm or become kinked.

Brachial artery injury results in peripheral ischaemia. The radius receives blood supply from collateral vessels. Median nerve damage results in loss of abduction of the thumb and loss of sensation over the thumb and lateral two and a half fingers. Median nerve injury tends to recover over a few weeks.

The axillary artery lies in the axilla and is not affected by low humeral damage.

Forearm oedema leads to 'compartment syndrome' and this leads to necrosis of the forearm muscles. Fasciotomy is required urgently.

Treatment options are:
- immobilisation in a sling
- closed reduction under general anaesthesia (GA)
- open reduction and fixation under GA.

Complications are:
- malunion
- non-union
- stiffness
- myositis ossificans

3.8   Gallstone ileus   Answers: B D

A complication of gallstones is inflammation of the gallbladder and ulceration into the adjacent duodenum. A cholecystoduodenal fistula results. Stones pass into the duodenum. Gas escapes into the biliary tree and this can be seen on abdominal X-ray.

A large stone passing into the duodenum obstructs the ileum, causing small bowel obstruction – this is gallstone ileus. Dilated small bowel is seen on an abdominal X-ray. Symptoms include colicky abdominal pain.

The large bowel has a larger calibre and the passage of stones is restricted by the ileocaecal valve. The large bowel therefore does not become obstructed. Symptoms tend to be colicky abdominal pain.

Treatment is by laparotomy and enterotomy to remove the obstructing stone. The cholecystoduodenal fistula is left in situ. Cholecystotomy is not required.

3.9   Blood transfusion   **Answers: A E**

Complications of blood transfusion include:

*   **febrile reaction** – this is due to release of pyrogens from cells and immune incompatibility. Pyrexia is a common occurrence and does not necessitate stopping the transfusion. However, if severe (> 38°C), transfusion should be stopped
*   **infections** transmitted by transfused blood include:
    *   viruses: hepatitis A, B, C and D (hepatitis B is screened by identification of the hepatitis B surface antigen but the problem with this is that it may be absent early after infection); HIV; HTLV; CMV; EBV.
    *   bacteria, eg syphilis
    *   others, eg malaria
*   **allergic reactions** manifest as pruritis, fever, rashes and angio-oedema
*   **haemolytic reactions** – haemolysis occurs in major ABO incompatibility, which is usually due to human error. Features are pyrexia, shortness of breath, loin pain, hypotension, acute renal failure, jaundice, disseminated intravascular coagulation.

3.10   A swelling with an expansile pulsation above the left clavicle
Answer: B

The key descriptions here are 'expansile pulsation' and the site, ie above the clavicle. A Pancoast tumour is a tumour of the lung occurring at the apex of the lung. The site is correct but the tumour would not have a pulsation.

The subclavian artery lies between the first rib and the clavicle. It can be tortuous or aneurysmal and this would cause it to be felt above the clavicle.

A cervical rib would exert pressure upwards, causing compression and narrowing. This results in stenosis: the symptoms include upper limb claudication on working with the arm above the head. The segment of artery beyond the stenosis becomes dilated (post-stenotic dilatation) and may form a thrombosis which may embolise, resulting in acute ischaemia.

The subclavian vein is not pulsatile.

Virchow's node is a painless enlarged lymph node in the left supraclavicular fossa, suggestive of gastric carcinoma. Palpation of a malignant node at this site is called 'Trosier's sign'.

A branchial cyst is a painless swelling in the side of the neck. The lump lies deep to the sternocleidomastoid muscle at the junction of its upper third and lower two-thirds. It presents in the anterior triangle of the neck. It is not pulsatile.

3.11   Ulcerative colitis   Answers: B D E

Ulcerative colitis presents with recurrent exacerbations of colonic inflammation. This causes diarrhoea, rectal bleeding and abdominal pain. It may lead to dehydration, fever, hypotension and tachycardia. Dilatation of the bowel may result in toxic megacolon and this may eventually perforate and cause peritonitis. Weight loss is common. Profuse diarrhoea with blood loss causes a fall in albumin. (See also Paper 1, Question 14; Paper 2, Question 48.)

3.12   Perforated peptic ulcer   Answers: A C D E

Perforation of a peptic ulcer is more commonly anterior than posterior. Duodenal ulcer perforation is more common than gastric ulcer perforation.

There may be a history of non-steroidal anti-inflammatory drug ingestion.

An erect chest X-ray shows gas under the diaphragm and this is detected clinically by resonance to percussion over the liver. It can be confirmed with a contrast study.

The typical presentation is of sudden-onset epigastric pain with vomiting.

There is rebound tenderness, guarding, board-like rigidity and cardiovascular collapse.

Posterior perforations tend to occur into the lesser sac which causes the peritonitis to remain localised.

3.13   Colonic polyps   **Answers: A B D**

A polyp is an abnormal growth of epithelium. It may be pedunculated (on a stalk) or sessile (broad-based and flat).

Adenoma describes a benign growth which appears tubular, villous or tubulovillous. In the large bowel all types are pre-malignant. The villous type has the greatest potential for malignant change and is usually sessile, whereas the tubular type has the least potential for malignant change and can be sessile or pedunculated. (The tubulovillous type lies in-between.)

Peutz–Jeghers syndrome is an autosomal dominant inherited condition. Numerous polyps occur in the small bowel. These are hamartomas and not adenomas. Spots of brown pigmentation may occur on the lips.

3.14   Crohn's disease   **Answers: A B E**

Crohn's disease and ulcerative colitis are inflammatory bowel diseases. Both are associated with clubbing. Crohn's disease affecting the small bowel may result in malabsorption of:

- iron ($\rightarrow$ iron deficiency anaemia) – absorbed in the duodenum
- vitamin B_{12} ($\rightarrow$ pernicious anaemia) – absorbed in the ileum
- folate – absorbed in the jejunum
- protein ($\rightarrow$ malnutrition)
- fat ($\rightarrow$ steatorrhoea)
- bile salts ($\rightarrow$ gallstone formation) – absorbed in the terminal ileum
- fat-soluble vitamins, ie vitamins A, D, E, K.

Crohn's disease commonly affects the terminal ileum, producing a 'terminal ileitis'. Inflammation results in narrowing. It affects the colon in about 25% of cases. It also affects the perianal region. The natural history is of chronic inflammatory disease with periods of relapse and remission.

3.15   Paralytic ileus   **Answers: A C E**

In paralytic ileus, the bowel is quiescent and there is a functional obstruction of the bowel. This results in dilatation of the bowel and vomiting. The signs are:

- inspection – abdominal distension
- palpation – tenderness which may be mild (or even absent)
- percussion – hyper-resonant
- auscultation – absent bowel sounds.

answers 3 Teaching 2 questions of

Colicky abdominal pain does not occur as there is no mechanical obstruction and the bowel is not contracting. X-rays show dilated loops of bowel with gas and fluid levels.

3.16 Dysphagia   Answers: A C D
Dysphagia is difficulty in swallowing. Do not confuse this with dysphasia which is impaired speech. Dysphagia occurs when there is an obstruction to the passage of solids or fluids in the oesophagus. Obstruction may be:
- in the lumen, eg carcinoma of the oesophagus
- in the oesophageal wall, eg benign stricture, carcinoma, pharyngeal pouch, leiomyoma
- outside the wall, eg carcinoma of the bronchus causing compression
- due to a disorder of motility, eg achalasia, stroke.

3.17 Diverticular disease   Answers: A C D
Diverticular disease is a common condition in Western society, caused by lack of fibre in the diet. It is asymptomatic. Inflammation of a diverticulum is 'diverticulitis'. It can occur in the small bowel but is far more common in the colon. It is not associated with malignancy. The complications and their presentations are listed below.

Complication	Presentations
Inflammation	Left iliac fossa pain
Inflammation/ haemorrhage	Rectal bleeding
Infection/sepsis/ abscess formation	Swinging pyrexia with abdominal pain
Perforation	'Rigid abdomen'
Fistulae	Pneumaturia
Stricture formation	Bowel obstruction with distension, vomiting etc

3.18   Femoral hernia   **Answers: B C E**

Although a truss may be useful, elective surgery for a femoral hernia is advised. It should be arranged at the earliest opportunity because femoral hernias have a high risk of strangulation.

Femoral hernias may contain omentum, fat, lymph nodes or bowel.

The anatomy is: femoral nerve; artery; vein; and femoral canal, from lateral to medial.

A femoral hernia appears below the inguinal ligament and lateral to the pubic tubercle.

Like any bowel hernia, it can strangulate without obstruction (see Paper 1, Question 18).

3.19   X-ray features of carcinoma of the colon versus diverticular disease   **Answers: A C D**

On a barium enema, carcinoma of the colon presents as an apple-core stricture, with shouldering.

Obstruction results in dilatation proximal to the stricture.

In contrast, diverticular disease is seen as numerous pockets – a saw-tooth appearance, which is due to numerous diverticula. A stricture in this case tends to affect a long segment of bowel and there may be spasm. Obstruction can also occur.

In both conditions, an abscess may appear as a gas bubble and if perforation occurs there may be gas under the diaphragm.

3.20   Acute cholecystitis   **Answers: A B D E**

Inflammation of the gallbladder may spread along the cystic and bile ducts towards the liver, causing ascending cholangitis, not cholecystitis (read the question carefully!). The inflammation may be chemical or it may be infective, due to *Escherichia coli* in the gastrointestinal tract.

If the gallbladder becomes infected it may fill with pus to form an empyema. Septicaemia may then ensue. Mucus secretion in the gallbladder may cause a mucocele which is palpable as an enlarged gallbladder.

Necrosis and gangrene may result in perforation of the gallbladder producing a peritonitis.

If the gallbladder perforates into a part of the bowel a cholecystoenteric fistula is created. Gallstones may then pass directly into the bowel and a gallstone ileus may result.

3.21   Hepatitis B
Answers: B C D

Hepatitis B virus is a DNA virus. It has an incubation period of two to six months. It is transmitted in blood products – by intravenous drug users, or in blood transfusions for example. Healthcare workers who are at risk of needlestick injuries or other injuries should be immunised with a course of three vaccinations. The clinical features include anorexia, malaise, nausea and vomiting. Jaundice and abdominal pain may occur. Liver function is affected and therefore clotting abnormalities may occur. Hepatitis B causes chronic hepatitis with an increased risk of cirrhosis and of hepatocellular carcinoma.

3.22   Ascending cholangitis
Answers: B C D E

Ascending cholangitis is characterised by pain, pyrexia and jaundice. Obstruction of the bile ducts due to gallstones, bile duct stricture or carcinoma predisposes to infection which ascends into the intrahepatic ducts. It may result in liver abscess. Invasive procedures, for example stent insertion, may introduce infection and cause cholangitis.

3.23   Carcinoma of the oesophagus
Answers: C D E

The classical presentation is dysphagia.

Investigations include a barium swallow; oesophagogastroduodenoscopy (OGD), which is very useful as biopsies can be taken if tumour is seen; and a CT scan, which is used to determine the extent of spread and to assess operability. Spread is local, to local lymph nodes and to the liver and lungs.

Radiotherapy is useful for squamous carcinoma.

Surgery is used for adenocarcinoma.

Chemotherapy is not used routinely.

3.24   Breast lump   **Answers: D E**

The skin changes in breast disease are often very marked. Tethering of the skin or dimpling is suggestive of carcinoma. Fixation to the skin or deeper tissues also suggests carcinoma. *Peau d'orange* is pathognomonic of carcinoma.

If a lump is present, its characteristics (ie surface and texture) provide useful information. Fibroadenoma usually produces a discrete lump with a smooth surface. It may be cystic. It is not fixed to the skin or deeper tissues. A lipoma is a soft mobile lump.

Intraductal papilloma is not usually felt as a lump and tends to present as nipple discharge.

An abscess affects the skin and subcutaneous tissue. It is red, hot and tender. Collection of pus makes it fluctuant and it may point and then discharge. It is fixed to the skin which may then become indurated.

Fat necrosis occurs following trauma to the breast. It forms a hard lump which may be fixed to the skin.

3.25   Splenic rupture   **Answers: A C D E**

A ruptured spleen presents with pain, tenderness and guarding in the left upper quadrant of the abdomen. Pain may be referred to the left shoulder. There is usually a history of trauma.

The signs of internal haemorrhage are:
- hypotension/hypovolaemia
- peritonitis, which may produce an ileus (if haemorrhage occurs into the peritoneal cavity)
- abdominal distension
- shifting dullness due to blood within the peritoneal cavity
- fixed dullness may occur due to extraperitoneal blood loss.

Haematemesis does not occur as bleeding is not within the bowel.

The diagnosis may be confirmed by ultrasound scan or CT scan.

Splenic rupture is treated by splenectomy with attention to vaccination and penicillin prophylaxis (see Paper 2, Question 8).

3.26 Renal calculi
Answers: B D E

Most renal calculi are idiopathic. The following factors predispose to their formation:

- stagnation of urine – congenital or acquired (obstruction)
- infection, eg urease-producing organisms such as *Proteus*
- dehydration/malnutrition
- raised calcium, eg, hyperparathyroidism, immobility
- gout – uric acid
- hyperoxaluria – calcium oxalate
- cysteinuria – cysteine stones.

3.27 Renal trauma
Answers: C D E

Injury to the kidney commonly results in localised pain and haematuria. Haematuria may be macroscopic or microscopic. Hypotension may occur. Appropriate investigations include:

- intravenous urogram
- ultrasound scan
- CT scan
- arteriography.

Treatment is usually conservative. Close monitoring of urine output, pulse rate and blood pressure is required.

The patient should be followed up for several months following renal trauma as complications such as hypertension or renal failure may develop late. There may be persistent bleeding. This may necessitate nephrectomy.

3.28 Ulcerative colitis
Answers: A C E

Ulcerative colitis is an inflammatory bowel disease (along with Crohn's disease, amoebiasis, etc) affecting the colon. The cause is unknown but genetic and environmental factors have been implicated.

It is a mucosal disease which involves the rectum and spreads proximally. There is inflammation of the mucosa, crypt abscesses and goblet cell depletion. Pseudopolyps occur where intact mucosa appears raised adjacent to ulcerated mucosa.

In patients with pancolitis the risk of malignancy is significant and total colectomy is advised.

3.29   Direct hernia   Answers: B C

Inguinal hernias occur above and medial to the pubic tubercle. A direct inguinal hernia is not controlled by pressure on the internal (deep) ring. An indirect inguinal hernia is controlled (after reduction) by pressure on the internal ring.

A direct inguinal hernia is due to weakness of the posterior wall of the inguinal canal such that the abdominal contents bulge forward. An indirect inguinal hernia is the passage of abdominal contents along the inguinal canal towards the scrotum. The two can occur together.

A direct inguinal hernia lies medial to the inferior epigastric vessels, whereas an indirect inguinal hernia lies lateral to them.

The risk of strangulation is low in a direct hernia.

3.30   Complications of venous insufficiency   Answers: A B C E

Chronic venous insufficiency causes:
* ankle flare due to venous hypertension
* dilated calf 'blow outs' due to incompetent valves
* superficial thrombophlebitis
* eczema
* pigmentation of the skin, usually over the medial aspect of the ankle; this may spread over the lower leg
* the skin may break down and ulcerate, especially over the medial malleolus; this may become infected and very painful; rarely, an ulcer undergoes malignant change, ie into a squamous cell carcinoma – this is called a Marjolin's ulcer
* lipodermatosclerosis may occur; the skin becomes red, hot and tender
* subcutaneous fibrosis causes stiffness of the ankle joint which may cause fixed flexion.

Venous insufficiency is a complication of deep vein thrombosis.

3.31   Digital gangrene   Answers: A C E

Digital gangrene is caused by obstruction of blood flow to the tips of the fingers. It occurs in peripheral arterial disease. The causes include:
* digital artery embolism, eg from the heart in atrial fibrillation or from a subclavian artery with atherosclerosis
* thrombus formation
* cervical rib: pressure on the sympathetic nerves may cause vasoconstriction; direct pressure on the subclavian artery would

reduce blood flow
- frostbite – where severe vasoconstriction causes hypoxia
- blood disorders, eg cold agglutinins
- vasculitis with vasospasm
- Raynaud's phenomenon
- drugs, eg ergot derivatives or β-blockers.

3.32   Pancreatitis   **Answers: C D**
The treatment of pancreatitis depends on the severity of the attack.

The patient is given intravenous fluids and kept 'nil by mouth'.

Antibiotics are given if there are signs of infection.

A nasogastric tube is inserted.

A urinary catheter is inserted to monitor urine output.

A central venous pressure (CVP) line may be required to control fluid balance.

Blood pressure and heart rate are monitored.

Analgesia is given as required.

For respiratory problems, oxygen is given via a mask; ventilation may be necessary. There is a risk of acute respiratory distress syndrome (ARDS).

Surgery is not the treatment of choice in acute pancreatitis.

The clinical picture in acute pancreatitis can be very deceptive.

In chronic pancreatitis, if the pancreatic tissue is severely damaged it is unable to mount a response and therefore a rise in serum amylase does not occur. Hence, a 'normal' amylase level can be seen when there is considerable pathology.

Other conditions which cause a rise in amylase include perforated peptic ulcer and trauma.

Essentially, the treatment is conservative. Laparotomy may be required for debridement of severe necrosis as a last resort.

3.33   Carbuncle   Answers: A C D E
A carbuncle is a widespread infection of the hair follicles and subcutaneous tissue caused by *Staphylococcus aureus*. It affects the adjacent skin and multiple sinuses develop. The back of the neck is commonly affected. It is more common in diabetics, hence the association with glycosuria. Treatment is with flucloxacillin.

3.34   Anal fissure   Answers: A D E
Definition: an anal fissure is a longitudinal tear of the anal mucosa. It is exquisitely painful and patients often refuse anorectal examination. Defecation causes pain with prolonged burning and impairs healing. The most common site is the posterior anal margin. It occurs in infants, children and adults.

Externally, there may be a skin tag called a 'sentinel pile'.

The anal sphincter may increase in tone causing constipation and bleeding which is detected as a smear on the toilet paper. There may also be pruritus.

Associated conditions are Crohn's disease, ulcerative colitis and tuberculosis.

3.35   Arterial embolus   Answers: A C D E
Definition: an embolus is the passage of a mass carried in the circulation. It produces its effects by lodging in smaller vessels and preventing oxygen and nutrients from reaching the tissues.

The different types of embolus include:
* thrombus – this is the most common
* fat – seen in fractures
* air – occurs in neck or lung trauma or iatrogenically
* nitrogen – caisson disease.

The management of emboli is:
* anticoagulation to prevent extension and recurrence
* thrombolysis – this is useful in patients in whom surgery is risky
* surgical embolectomy.

The site of origin varies – commonly it arises in the heart and is caused by atrial fibrillation. It is the site where the embolus lodges rather than its site of origin that determines its effects. The size of the embolus will determine the site of impact and therefore its effects. The main effect of an embolus is ischaemia. The presence of a collateral circulation may therefore allow the tissue to remain viable.

An infected embolus, for example an embolus of vegetations from the heart, can lodge in an artery and cause a mycotic aneurysm.

3.36   Coronary artery bypass graft   Answer: D
Coronary artery surgery may be performed on or off cardiopulmonary bypass. It is performed using the left internal mammary artery or a saphenous vein. Three- or four-vessel disease produces marked symptoms and hence surgery is very successful in relieving symptoms.

Investigations required prior to operation include:
*   chest X-ray
*   electrocardiogram (ECG)
*   exercise ECG
*   coronary angiography.

The operative mortality is 2–3%. In addition to the general complications, specific complications include strokes, neurological deficit and graft failure.

Surgery provides:
*   reduced morbidity with relief of symptoms in most cases
*   reduced mortality.

In patients with three- or four-vessel disease and severe symptoms, such as unstable angina, the mortality is reduced following operation. However, in patients with one- or two-vessel disease, mortality is not improved by the operation.

3.37   Deep vein thrombosis (DVT) prophylaxis   Answers: A B C
There is a significant risk of DVT post-operatively.

Predisposing factors include trauma, surgery, dehydration, immobilisation, malignancy, polycythaemia and the oral contraceptive pill. The risk is higher following major operations.

Measures used to prevent DVT are:
- minimal trauma to the legs during handling of the patient
- rehydration – increased blood viscosity predisposes to thrombosis
- heparin (subcutaneous, 5000 IU twice daily)
- elasticated compression stockings
- pneumatic calf stockings during operations
- early mobilisation
- warfarin – but there is a risk of haemorrhage
- intravenous dextran.

3.38   Surgical emphysema   Answers: B D

Surgical emphysema is caused by air tracking into subcutaneous tissues. Clinically there is swelling of the affected area with crepitus. It may be visible on X-ray.

The causes are trauma and oesophageal rupture. Treatment is of the underlying cause. The surgical emphysema itself tends to resolve.

3.39   Anal pain   Answers: A C E

Lesions in the anal canal can present with pain.

Carcinoma can cause ulceration with bleeding and pain.

Perianal haematoma causes a localised inflammatory reaction which is painful.

Haemorrhoids are not painful *per se*, but it is their complications which cause pain; first-degree haemorrhoids are internal and not painful.

Anal warts cause irritation and discomfort; they do not produce pain. Anal fissure is classically very painful, as can be fistula-in-ano, especially when infection occurs.

A perianal abscess causes pain and discomfort, especially on sitting.

3.40   Malignant melanoma   Answers: B D E

Most malignant melanomas arise in normal skin. Only a minority arise in a pre-existing mole. The prognosis depends on depth of invasion. There are two classification systems used to determine prognosis:
- **Clark's level** of invasion is based on the layer of skin penetrated – if the basement membrane is not penetrated the prognosis is good; invasion into the subcutaneous fat carries a very poor prognosis.

- **Breslow's classification** uses the thickness of the tumour ('Breslow's index') to predict prognosis:

Depth of invasion (mm)	Risk
< 0.76	Low
0.76–1.5	Moderate
> 1.5	High

Most lesions are of the superficial spreading type. These have a better prognosis than the nodular type which invade deeply.

Amelanotic lesions have a worse prognosis. This may be because they are diagnosed late or because they are inherently more aggressive.

Malignant melanomas spread via lymphatics to the regional lymph nodes, and via the bloodstream to the lungs, liver and brain.

3.41 Peripheral arterial disease   Answers: A B D E
Intermittent claudication is a sign of chronic lower limb ischaemia. As this worsens it develops into rest pain and critical ischaemia. Critical ischaemia is arterial disease which threatens the viability of the foot or leg. It usually occurs gradually but can develop suddenly if there is thrombus or embolus occluding a vessel.

In acute critical ischaemia of the foot the classic features are the six 'P's:
  Pain
  Pallor
  Pulseless
  Paraesthesia (numbness of the foot)
  Paralysis (this is a late sign)
  Perishing with cold

Transient ischaemic attacks are a feature of ischaemic events in the brain which may result from carotid artery emboli.

Diabetes mellitus is associated with atherosclerosis. However, it is not a feature of peripheral arterial disease. Also, diabetic neuropathy results in injury and ulceration of the feet due to poor healing.

3.42   Tuberculosis   Answers: B C D E

The incidence of tuberculosis (TB) is increasing in the UK. It is caused by *Mycobacterium tuberculosis* which can affect the lungs, bones, gastrointestinal tract, urinary tract and skin. It is characterised by granuloma formation and caseating necrosis. Pus forms slowly and results in the formation of an abscess. As the abscess forms slowly and there is no redness/inflammation, it is called a 'cold abscess'.

Infection of the spine can be devastating. It affects both the bone and the intervertebral disc spaces. Vertebral collapse may cause spinal cord compression which requires surgical intervention.

TB spreads via the bloodstream to the genitourinary tract. Tuberculous epididymitis causes swelling of the scrotum, but symptoms may be mild and go unnoticed.

TB affecting the urinary tract causes frequency of micturition as is seen in bacterial urinary tract infection.

3.43   Carcinoma of the tongue   Answers: C E

Carcinoma of the tongue occurs most commonly on the anterior two-thirds of the tongue. It is more common in men than women. There is an association with pipe smoking, alcohol, leukoplakia, betel nut chewing and poor oral hygiene.

The presentation is of a nodule or ulcer. The tongue is covered in squamous epithelium and therefore the carcinoma is squamous in type. Spread occurs locally or by lymphatic drainage to the sub-mental and cervical lymph nodes.

Prognosis depends on spread. If metastasis has occurred, the five-year survival rate is only 18%.

Definitive treatment is by surgery, radiotherapy or both.

3.44   Prolapsed lumbar disc   Answers: B C D E

A prolapsed lumbar disc classically presents with back pain radiating to the buttock. There may be paraesthesia of the leg and muscle weakness.

At the affected level, reflexes are diminished, for example, L3/4 – knee jerk; L5/S1 – ankle jerk. Cauda equina compression may cause urinary retention.

Treatment of a prolapsed disc is by the three 'R's:
   Rest
   Removal
   Rehabilitation

Improvement may occur following rest alone.

3.45 Bone metastases   Answers: A C E
This is a list well worth committing to memory. Tumours commonly metastasising to bone include:

* breast
* thyroid
* bronchus
* prostate – remember that this causes sclerotic lesions
* kidney.

Lesions are lytic (except prostate) and present as pathological fractures.

3.46 Heparin   Answer: C
Heparin inhibits blood coagulation by inactivation of thrombin and coagulation factors VII, IX, X, XI and XII. Intermittent subcutaneous injection is given for prophylaxis of venous thrombosis (5000 IU twice daily). Intravenous therapy is given for the treatment of deep vein thrombosis.

Heparin has a short half-life of about one hour. It is reversible with protamine. The best test for monitoring therapy is the activated partial thromboplastin time (APTT).

The international normalised ratio (INR) is a measure of the prothrombin time which is used to monitor warfarin activity.

Long-term heparin therapy causes osteoporosis, not osteomalacia

3.47 Intertrochanteric fracture of the femur   Answers: B C
Intertrochanteric fractures of the femur occur in the elderly, especially in women who have osteoporosis, which weakens the bones. The fracture may be traumatic or pathological. The classic presentation is shortening of the leg and external rotation.

Intertrochanteric fractures are extracapsular. Therefore, they unite early with little risk of avascular necrosis. Treatment is by internal fixation to allow early mobilisation.

3.48   Antibiotics   **Answers: A D E**

Antibiotics are often used to prevent infection in surgery. A short sharp dosage is recommended (ie 1–3 doses given intravenously). Prolonged courses are not advantageous. The definitive treatment of an abscess is incision and drainage. Patients at high risk of infection during surgery require prophylactic antibiotics, for example patients with prosthetic heart valves, rheumatic heart disease, etc.

Cefuroxime (a second-generation cephalosporin) is active against enterococci and is often used for prophylaxis in cholecystectomy. In colorectal surgery, the major risk of infection is due to bowel organisms, ie anaerobes – metronidazole is used for this. A cephalosporin is added for prophylaxis against aerobes.

3.49   Complications of urinary catheter insertion   **Answers: C D E**

The passage of a urinary catheter presents a risk of infection both on insertion and removal. Epithelial damage allows access for bacteria into the circulation and septicaemia can result.

Artificial prostheses are particularly at risk. It is thus very important to use aseptic technique.

Antibiotic cover (eg, gentamicin intramuscularly) can be used. Trauma during insertion may cause urethral bleeding.

Trauma to the prostate gland can cause acute prostatitis.

Renal calculi and chronic pyelonephritis are not a problem.

3.50   Hyperhidrosis   **Answers: D E**

Hyperhidrosis is excess sweating of the skin. It is a common complaint and can be very distressing when it occurs in the hands. It classically occurs in young women. The aetiology is unknown but it is thought to be due to excessive vasomotor activity, via sympathetic nerves. Treatment includes:

*   axillary skin excision – the hair-bearing area containing sweat glands is removed as a thin layer of skin
*   cervical sympathectomy, used to abolish palmar sweating; a recognised complication of this is Horner's syndrome
*   lumbar sympathectomy, used to abolish sweating of the soles.

3.51   Pre-operative investigations   Answers: A B E
The urgent investigations required in large bowel obstruction are:
- full blood count
- urea and electrolytes
- creatinine
- chest X-ray
- ECG.

These are the minimum requirements to facilitate safe anaesthesia.

Sigmoidoscopy is unlikely to alter the management.
A barium enema would cause delay. Laparotomy would still be required
to relieve the obstruction.

3.52   Pseudomembranous colitis   Answers: B C D
Pseudomembranous colitis is colitis due to antibiotic therapy. Clindamycin
was one of the first antibiotics to be implicated but cephalosporin therapy
is more common. Pseudomembranous colitis is caused by an overgrowth
of *Clostridium difficile*. It causes a profound watery diarrhoea and the
formation of a membrane on the intestinal mucosa. Investigation is by:
- sigmoidoscopy and biopsy
- detection of *Clostridium difficile* toxin in the stool
- culture of *Clostridium difficile* from the stool.

Treatment is oral metronidazole or oral vancomycin.

3.53   Earl post-operative complications   Answers: A C D E
In the first 12 hours after an operation, complications are either those due
to anaesthesia or those due to the surgery.

Complications of anaesthesia include:
- drug reactions or side-effects
- trauma to the mouth or throat
- post-operative nausea and vomiting
- fluid imbalance: a fluid chart is essential to monitor fluid input and
  output. Bowel surgery causes loss of large amounts of fluid and
  hypovolaemia may result – this predisposes to acute renal failure. If
  excess fluid is given, cardiac failure may occur due to overloading
- hypothermia – this can occur in bowel surgery where fluid loss is
  high and operations are long
- lung atelectasis/aspiration: hypoxia may result and therefore
  attention must be paid to oxygenation.

Complications of surgery include reactionary haemorrhage. Wound drainage is used to monitor any internal blood loss.

(See also Paper 2, Question 51.)

3.54   Total parenteral nutrition (TPN)   Answers: B D
TPN is intravenous feeding; enteral nutrition is feeding via the gastro-intestinal tract.

TPN is indicated for malnourished patients in whom the gastrointestinal tract is not functioning, for example in obstruction.

Pre-operatively, TPN is beneficial for patients who are severely malnourished, ie only about 5% of patients.

Post-operatively, TPN is beneficial in malnourished patients as it improves wound healing and is required to overcome the catabolic phase.

TPN solutions have high osmolalities and are therefore highly thrombophlebitic. They are therefore given via a central venous line into large veins where blood flow is high. The risks of central venous line insertion include haemorrhage, pneumothorax, air embolism and sepsis.

Enteral feeding is usually given via a fine-bore nasogastric tube. If this is not tolerated, a percutaneous endoscopic gastrostomy (PEG) can be used.

3.55   Rectal bleeding   Answers: A B D
Bleeding per rectum occurs in:
* diverticulitis
* carcinoma of the rectum or colon
* haemorrhoids
* Meckel's diverticulum
* intussusception
* colitis – blood and mucus are seen
* melaena – old dark blood from peptic ulceration.

Intussusception occurs when a segment of bowel 'telescopes' into the adjacent section. It is most common before the age of two years. Ileo-caecal intussusception is the most common form. It presents with bowel obstruction and the blood passed per rectum is described as 'redcurrant jelly stool' and is pathognomonic. The management is urgent barium enema which confirms the diagnosis and may even relieve the intussusception – if not, laparotomy is required.

Carcinoma of the oesophagus presents with faecal occult blood, but not blood on digital examination.

3.56   Thyroid carcinoma   Answers: A B D
Thyroid carcinoma is divided into four types:
* papillary
* follicular
* anaplastic
* medullary.

Papillary carcinoma affects children and young adults, females more than males. It presents as a slow-growing lump. It is slow to spread and does so via lymphatics. It may therefore present with enlargement of lymph nodes. It moves on swallowing and is not fixed to the skin. There is an association with previous radiation. The standard treatment is total thyroidectomy and the prognosis is excellent.

Follicular carcinoma affects adults aged 40–50 years. It spreads via the bloodstream to lungs and bones and may therefore present with shortness of breath or bone pain. Treatment is thyroid lobectomy; if metastases are present total thyroidectomy is performed.

Anaplastic tumours present in older patients, aged 60–80 years. It is more common in women than men. Spread is rapid. Patients present with a hard thyroid lump and symptoms of local invasion, such as hoarseness if the recurrent laryngeal nerve is affected, or stridor if the trachea is compressed. The prognosis is worse in this type. Surgical treatment is palliative.

Medullary carcinoma is a well-differentiated carcinoma of parafollicular cells, which secrete calcitonin. It affects patients aged 50–70 years. The treatment is total thyroidectomy.

Thyroid carcinomas do **not** usually cause thyroid dysfunction. Patients are often euthyroid.

3.57   Transplant surgery   **Answers: B C D E**

Renal transplantation has increased in numbers and success. It is used for patients in chronic renal failure and end-stage renal failure. Consideration is given to the patient's condition; patients over the age of 50 years are not excluded.

Transfer of tissue (for example, skin from one part of the body to another) is an **autograft**; from person to person is an **allograft**; from one species to another is a **xenograft**.

Rejection is due to the presence of antibodies and is a major problem. Prevention is by tissue typing and immunosuppression.

Any infection must be treated prior to surgery.

3.58   Bowel stricture   **Answers: B C D**

Bowel stricture is caused by a local inflammatory response.

The causes include:
*   diverticular disease
*   neoplasia
*   Crohn's disease
*   mesenteric ischaemia
*   slow-release potassium tablets.

Peutz–Jeghers syndrome is a cause of intestinal polyposis.

3.59   Amylase   **Answers: A C D E**

A marked rise in serum amylase occurs in acute pancreatitis (> 1000 IU/l). However, the level is not indicative of severity. Other causes include:
*   diabetic ketoacidosis
*   perforated peptic ulcer (not > 400 IU/l)
*   acute cholecystitis
*   renal failure
*   strangulated bowel.

Acute appendicitis does not cause raised amylase.

3.60   Volvulus   **Answers: A B C**
Volvulus is a twisting of a loop of bowel. It usually occurs in the elderly
and presents with abdominal distension and pain. Constipation may also
be present. Complications are venous infarction or perforation resulting in
peritonitis.

Investigations include a plain abdominal X-ray which shows a dilated
bowel – the sigmoid colon is commonly affected and has an inverted
horseshoe appearance.

The treatment is:
- insertion of a flatus tube
- barium enema without preparation
- surgery – laparotomy, sigmoid colectomy.

MCQ REVISION INDEX

The numbers after each entry refer to the examination and question number.

MCQ Revision Index

RECOMMENDED READING LIST

An Introduction to the Signs and Symptoms of Surgical Disease 3rd edition
Norman Browse, Hodder Arnold, 1997.

Essential Surgery: Problems, Diagnosis and Management 3rd edition
George Burkitt et al, Churchill Livingstone, 2001.

Lecture Notes on General Surgery 10th edition
Harold Ellis, Blackwell Science (UK), 2002.

Surgical Finals: Passing the Clinical 2nd edition
John Lumley & Gina Kuperberg, PasTest, 2003.

PASTEST REVISION BOOKS

PasTest are the specialists in study guides and revision courses for professional medical qualifications. For over 30 years we have been helping doctors to achieve their potential. The new PasTest range of books for medical students includes:

Essential MCQs for Medical Finals, Second edition
Rema Wasan, Delilah Hassanally, Balvinder Wasan   ISBN 1 901198 20 0

Essential MCQs in Clinical Pharmacology
Delilah Hassanally, Rema Singh   ISBN 1 901198 32 4

EMQs for Medical Students Volume 1
Adam Feather et al   ISBN 1 901198 65 0

EMQs for Medical Students Volume 2
Adam Feather et al   ISBN 1 901198 69 3

OSCEs for Medical Undergraduates Volume 1
Adam Feather, Ramanathan Visvanathan,   ISBN 1 901198 04 9
John SP Lumley

OSCEs for Medical Undergraduates Volume 2
Ramanathan Visvanathan, Adam Feather,   ISBN 1 901198 05 7
John SP Lumley

Medical Finals: Passing the Clinical
Christopher Moore, Anne Richardson   ISBN 1 901198 43 6

Surgical Finals: Passing the Clinical, Second edition
John SP Lumley, Gina Kuperberg   ISBN 1 901198 77 4

Medical Finals: Structured Answers and Essay Questions
Adam Feather, Ramanathan Visvanathan,   ISBN 1 901198 79 7
John SP Lumley

Surgical Finals: Structured Answers and Essay Questions
Ramanathan Visvanathan, John SP Lumley   ISBN 1 901198 43 X

Learning by Lists for Medical Students
Stuart McPherson   ISBN 1 901198 30 8

The Practical Guide to Medical Ethics and Law for Junior Doctors and Medical Students
Chloe-Maryse Baxter, Mark Brennan, Yvette Coldicott ISBN 1 901198 76 6

Radiology Casebook for Medical Students
Rema Wasan, Alan Grundy, Richard Beese   ISBN 1 901198 40 5

Clinical Skills for Medical Students: A Hands-on Guide
Ian Bickle, David McCluskey, Barry Kelly   ISBN 1 901198 86 3

Essential MCQs in Obstetrics and Gynaecology for Medical Students
Diana Hamilton-Fairley   ISBN 1 901198 34 0